Closing Comments

ALS—a Spiritual Journey into the Heart of a Fatal Affliction

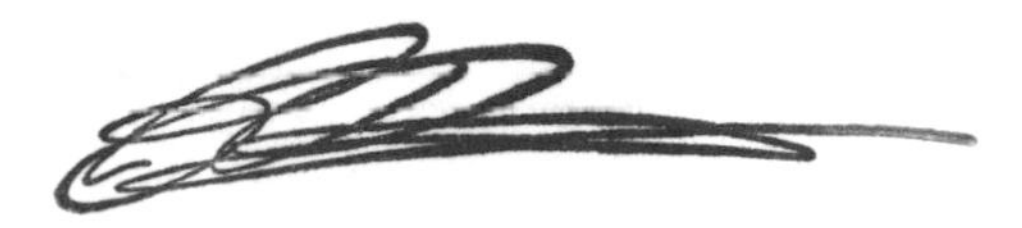

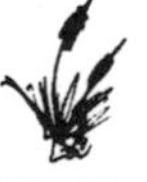

CLEMENTS PUBLISHING
Toronto

#104, 3373 Capilano Crescent
North Vancouver, BC
V7R 4W7 Canada
E-mail: blsmith@telus.net

First edition

Published 2000 by Clements Publishing
Box 213, 6021 Yonge Street
Toronto, ON
M2M 3W2 Canada
Website: www.clementspublishing.com

Design and typesetting by Greg Reimer, g&L Page Design

Printed in Canada

A cataloguing record for this publication is available from the National Library of Canada

ISBN 1-894667-06-9

Contents

Foreword v
Introduction vii

Embracing the Ambiguities of Life 1
Looking for Ways to Escape 18
The Perilous Path of Romance 32
Ominously Hopeful Symptoms 49
Someone Else will Carry You 60
Never the Same Again 69
Springtime and Fall Laced Together 77
Laughing and Crying My Way to Heaven 88
Getting to the Wedding on Time 106
Closing Comments 118

Eulogy by Wally Eggert 124
At the Graveside 134
Chronology 139

Foreword

In January 1996 Brian and I were in Cyprus. Brian brought with him Annie Dillard's book *An American Childhood.* It was a gift for the journey from his niece, Tracey. We would sit in the sun, in sheltered places, and he would read me bits. His eyes would fill with tears. He loved the content, but it was the way that Dillard crafted a sentence that moved him so. I fell ever more deeply in love with this man who would become my husband.

Brian always loved beautifully crafted things. It was not uncommon for him to stop in front of a well-made stone wall or a man-made waterfall and admire it. He had great admiration for good craftsmanship. He would sit in his chair looking out the window of our home and watch his favourite Towhee hop around the bushes, head up, calling out. He loved the supreme creator and craftsman who had created such wonderful birds. As Brian's health declined and he was no longer able to craft with wood and stone he turned his creative craftsman's heart to writing.

Brian wrote for his family, friends and himself. He wanted to leave something tangible for those he loved so dearly. This past summer, Paul Stevens, a friend of many years, read

Brian's work, declared it good and encouraged him to keep writing.

As you read this I know you will laugh and cry as we have done for the past few years. I hope you will come away encouraged in faith and hope. This is Brian's gift to us.

Lynne Smith
November 6, 2000

> *Therefore we do not lose heart. Though outwardly we are wasting away, yet inwardly we are being renewed day by day. For our light and momentary troubles are achieving for us an eternal glory that far outweighs them all. So we fix our eyes not on what is seen, but on what is unseen. For what is seen is temporary, but what is unseen is eternal (2 Corinthians 4:16–18).*

Introduction: Superman in a Power Chair

In a physical sense I have become almost powerless. It is dangerous for me to stand without someone near me. I am limited to four or five steps, with something to hold on to, before I am completely out of breath. My diaphragm has weakened to the point where I have less than 35 percent lung capacity so that minimal physical activity such as brushing my teeth exhausts me.

The days wound down to the sixtieth birthday extravaganza that Lynne had so carefully planned for me on the twenty-ninth of last month. We expected 130 people to attend this glorious event, at which I had planned to make a power chair grand entrance wearing my Superman suit, under the forceful cadence of The Village People singing "Macho Man."

Afterwards, I would slowly recover from 130 short conversations sprinkled through the excitement of a great night. The party was a smash. My friend, Gord Taylor, was magnificent as M.C. and all supporting cast members performed admirably. My son, Kyle, prepared all the music including a THX opening crescendo prior to "Macho Man." I rode in to thunderous ovation, circled the dance floor in my chair with a couple of extra twirls, and moved to the mike to welcome my guests. Many of them had not seen me since I was doing some walking and so they were seeing me in a chair for the first time. Attempting to make reference to the skeletal frame in the Superman suit, which had only the few years earlier performed its own stunts, I said "Well, that was one hell of a piece of kryptonite." Reasonable laughter followed, and then I said, "Thank you all for coming to my sixtieth. The Bible says a natural lifespan is three score and ten years. I, at least, have three score. That's one score more than I made with women. On with the show!"

In keeping with the Superman entrance we had obtained a copy of a video taken at the family camp that Barb, my first wife, and I had directed over the years and where the Superman suit gained its notoriety. This particular episode related to a series of videos prepared by some of the kids at camp, titled "Bathrooms of the Rich and Famous." Following this theme we arranged to have the kids track down Superman to determine what his bathroom looked like. The image needs to be seen to be appreciated but Superman runs to a tree where he reaches down under the cover of his cape and begins to pee. The stream actually comes from a hose with a narrowed nozzle hidden by the tree and started by signal. Superman somehow allows the furious jet of water to hit the tree and spray all over himself. The effect of this video, replayed at my sixtieth, was quite startling and received 260 thumbs up from the crowd. It was a splendid start to the festivities. Today, of course, Superman cannot even put on his own undershorts.

As dessert commenced Gord announced that the mike was open for lies, exaggerations, pre-fabrications and even true stories. About a dozen people accommodated with their accounts of various episodes in my life and I closed this session with a brief monologue that went something like this:

> *Nothing like a great party to end your day. The other day a friend asked me what my daily routine was like. I said that my daily routine has been pretty much the same for all of my life. I get up in the morning much sooner than I would like to and I go to bed at night later than I should. In between time I keep asking myself the question, "How did I get into this mess?"*

That was April 29, 2000.

My story begins right now. It starts now because my friend, Jim, smiled at me over the folds of his blanket and lipped the silent words, "Get going." I had been asking him about his efforts at putting his story to words and mourning my own lack of discipline to do the same. He wasn't telling me to leave his hospital room. He was telling me to get my butt in gear. Well, maybe not my butt; it lost its gears long ago. He was really referring to my left index finger, the only appendage I have left with a modicum of dexterity. With it, a microphone and a computer, I too can tell my story.

Jim and I have formed a friendship out of mutual anguish. We both have Amyotrophic Lateral Sclerosis (ALS), a rapidly progressive neuromuscular disease. It attacks the motor neurons that transmit electrical impulses from the brain to the voluntary muscles in the body. When these muscles fail to receive messages they lose strength, atrophy and die. ALS does not affect the mind or senses. In 90 percent of cases it strikes people with no family history of the disease. Jim had been in the hospital for two months trying to adjust to being attached to a respirator while fighting infection and various other manifestations of this trying disorder. I was visiting, riding my high-tech, even-terrain vehicle and seeing myself mirrored in this hospital scene some unknown number of months down the road.

Of course, stories don't begin right now. They only come to mind in the present; they are built on the past and continue in the future. We write about our past and speculate on the future. Though with this disease, there is less speculation. Options narrow and the future becomes much more certain—a kind of certainty that is deadly and that tends to bring the past into focus.

But this is not my first experience at narrowing options and deadly certainties.

Embracing the Ambiguities of Life

"Death is not a breaker but a renewer of ties."
George MacDonald

Barb was busy as usual with hospitality but approaching the magic year when her own mother had died of a dread disease. Otherwise the final decade of the millennium began peacefully for my family and me. Four children were healthily progressing in various stages of life. Our two oldest boys, ages 20 and 22, were happily engaged in construction trades. Our daughter, fifteen, was drifting through high school as if it were a social calendar, while our youngest son, 12, was entering puberty with a grin on his unsuspecting face. And I had finally escaped from a financial nightmare that had taken up a substantial chunk of my energies in the '80s. Life seemed to be filled with endless possibilities.

The "C" Word is Back

It was in October of 1993 that the accumulating force of life changing events made me realize that sometimes possibilities can be limited and settling into my computer chair I wrote:

It's back! The "C" word once again demands its place in the lexicon of our lives. My urge to write almost meshed with my need to emote when it came the first time. But it seems that when things that are ugly come back the second time they're stronger than the first and so with a violent blend of literary urge and fear I launch this chronicle of an unknown path.

November '91. Barb's tears rippled through the phone, and mixed with the words, "I have cancer in my bowel," made me realize in an instant that something was finished and something else was starting. Now almost two years later, though the year between the completion of chemo and start of the back and leg pains was a bit of back to normal, the "something else" has resumed.

A client had invited me to play golf earlier in the week and I said yes. And though I knew there was a chance that the roof of our lives that had sprung a leak two years ago might fall in on us today, I went. I thought of cancelling this morning so I would be with her, but I rationalized that more than likely the result would be negative and I would have wasted my day worrying about it. I didn't get home until after Barb had gone to work.

We fried chicken, boiled peas and made some toast for dinner and settled in to watch the Jays get pounded by the Sox. I couldn't face work, which is where I should have gone. A little reading, a little kitchen cleaning and wasp flushing (each day a new batch of wasps come up through the holes in the floor of our partly renovated bathroom from their paper maché dormitory in our crawl space to expend the tiny limit of their lives in the deadly cul-de-sac of the skylight) and a little more TV watching, killed the time to 11:15 p.m., Barb's ETA.

I didn't ask when she arrived. Fraser, our 14-year-old son, had no idea of the implications of the test, or maybe even that there had been one, and, without knowing, could get one more night without having any of this marring his sleep. So, as we got into bed, I asked.

Soon, life as I had known it was fading away in the transparent community of affliction and death as friends and family, spreading sympathy and support, created an atmosphere of blended cheer and gloom at home and hospital. My wife of 28 years was in the final days of her productive and creative life and we and our four children were centre stage in life's most certain drama.

So it is with some personal experience of affliction and death that I attempt to express some thoughts on how we might tolerate these unwelcome crusaders which turn our personal ambitions and goals to dimly lit and quickly fading dreams. Are these challenges an obstacle to or an opportunity for holy living? How does holy living contend with affliction, disease and death?

Round two for Barb was shorter than round one. A common encomium ascribed to losers in the battle with terminal illness is the frequently used phrase, "after a valiant battle." But I couldn't say she battled. She was more like a cork on the sea, moved from one wave to the next by another medical manipulation. Up one side with more painkillers and down the other side with another advance by the enemy—that was her story, always perilously close to the rocks. There is no battle here, only motion, and that by some invisible force. Barb died on August 11, 1994, quietly acquiescing to the inevitable. Meanwhile, unknown to me, some other variant of the genetic forces that control our earthly destiny was already expressing itself in my brain and spinal cord. My cork was farther at sea, and following more gradual currents, but, nonetheless, moving closer to the uncertainties of the shore.

At the memorial a friend provided a eulogy suggesting that we had "done it well." But I wonder. How can you do this "well"? Maybe it was really Barb who had done it well. She never complained about her lot, she just quietly accepted the inevitable, wrote letters of encouragement to her children and slipped slowly out of misery into mystery. Possibly "doing it well" for those who watch is just to keep on loving the one you are losing and each other as well. There are two stages in this process and both involve hope. From the onset of illness you have hope for recovery. In a way that hope continues to the end but somewhere realism interferes and hope for something beyond takes its place.

The Family Spiritual Inheritance

We face our hurdles with a toolbox full of our history. We can end up with the right tools or the wrong tools in our hands. They can be rusty or well-oiled, but they are all we have. I think I am fortunate in having a toolbox full of well-oiled and usable utensils. One of them is the history of faith. I was the second of four children born to Allen and Phoebe Smith. My Dad was the oldest of thirteen children born to Noble and Bertha Smith on a rock-infested quarter section of homestead land near Gladstone, Manitoba. I have not researched the history of their religious beliefs but somehow they became part of a Protestant denomination known as the Plymouth Brethren. So when my father moved to Vancouver in his twenties he was able to make connections with a related church. My mother was one of three children born to Gertrude Adamson, whose dramatic and uncompromising conversion to Christianity drove her husband from his home, leaving her to raise the children alone, unencumbered by an unbelieving spouse. For economic reasons my mother left school after grade eight to work as a clerk in Spencer's department store. Her adherence to the Christian faith resulted in the marital union which ultimately caused my spirit to rise from the place to which my inherited, but personally accepted faith, says it will return. So it was my destiny to be infected by the supernatural scope of Scripture and to increasingly rely upon it for comfort and direction. And a handy tool it has been.

> *"The LORD brought me forth as the first of his works, before his deeds of old; I was appointed from eternity, from the beginning, before the world began. When there were no oceans, I was given birth, when there were no springs abounding with water; before the mountains were settled in place, before the hills, I was given birth, before he made the earth or its fields or any of the dust of the world. I was there when he set the heavens in place, when he marked out the horizon on the face of the deep, when he established the clouds above and fixed securely the fountains of the deep, when he gave the sea its boundary so the waters would not overstep his command, and when he marked out the foundations of the earth. Then I was the craftsman at his side. I was filled with delight day after day, rejoicing always in his presence, rejoicing in his whole world and delighting in mankind" (Proverbs 8:22–31).*

My earliest memories of thumbing the pages of a Bible were in the musty Sunday School rooms of Central Park

Gospel Hall, an example of the simplest church architecture ever dedicated to the Lord for worship. But it had remarkable flexibility. Aside from the basement, which could be sectioned into several rooms by curtains, the two cloak rooms at the entrance, rooms on either side of the preaching platform, and two rooms in the apex of the roof above the entrance, provided ample space for various grades. There was no written material other than the Bible and the teaching method was normally to read and talk while the musing minions shuffled their feet and looked anxiously at the clock on the wall which was always heading towards lunch time. Hands-on Bible study in Sunday School was only one of three opportunities each Sunday to hear what the Scripture could offer the inquiring, or distracted, mind.

Memories of Sunday

Sunday was a full day for Plymouth Brethren. It started at 9:00 a.m. with "the breaking of bread service," a quaint alternative terminology for "communion." The classic wooden dowelled chairs were placed in a quadrangle facing the centrally located communion table. A white linen tablecloth and napkins covering the sacred elements provided a modest sense of a sacredness to the otherwise artless decor. A quiet exchange of greetings at the top of the entrance stairs as hymn books were handed to the worshipers and the creaking of the oiled fir floor were the only sounds to be heard other than the gentle ticking of the clock.

There was an established ritual to the event. Within seconds of the scheduled start one of the men, familiar with the routine, would announce a hymn, carefully reading the first verse allowing everyone time to find it in the book. Then, with no musical accompaniment, the appointed key and melody setter would start singing solo with everyone slowly joining the chorus. Each hymn had a series of numbers strung out under the heading, which had some mysterious relationship to chords or melody. Once things were underway any of the men, assumed to be led by the Holy Spirit, would pray, read a Scripture, or indulge in a short or lengthy discourse on a selected passage. Eventually, within an acceptable but unstated time slot, somewhere around the 40-minute mark, someone would give thanks in his prayer for the broken bread and an elder would quietly move towards the table, remove the napkin, break the bread into two pieces and start the distribution on silver plates. In a similar manner the wine would be served, the offering bags passed and with a concluding hymn and announcements a gentle growing chatter would emanate from the faithful as they slowly moved towards the door.

Somehow money was always found in our tight budget to present ourselves at this solemn service attired in suits and Sunday dresses. The ritual of eating and dressing on Sunday morning rarely started early enough to get us to the church on time, so there was invariably blame being pointed in several directions over who had caused the delays. Tension would often be high as we sped through the early morning traffic hoping like heck that the Holy Spirit would hold everybody off long enough for us to get to our front row seats before the first hymn was finished. Arriving during the hymn was bad enough but getting there after the hymn meant that the sounds of two adults and four children creeping down the aisle and sliding into their seats would reverberate unmercifully among the turning heads. My mother, mortified by this demeaning performance, would refuse to raise her head until about the third hymn while her hat, an obligatory symbol of deference to men, was tilted to hide her flushing face. In spite of the disgrace that this procedure heaped upon her, my mother was unable to exert sufficient influence upon her husband and children to consistently avoid it. To this day, when I see her suffering from Alzheimer's disease, slouched in her wheelchair peering vacantly up at me through her wispy bangs, I think I can still see the shame in her eyes.

As a breakaway movement from the Church of England, the Brethren had an aversion to most common terminologies. We didn't go to "church." We were an "Assembly." But the most fundamental aversion was to any scent of professionalism from the pulpit. "Pastor," "Father" and "Priest" were words not found in the New Testament in the context of leadership. "Pastoring" was a spiritual gift, not an office; "Father," a word that could be ascribed only to God; and we were all "priests," giving rise to the catch phrase and the fundamental tenet of the way we did things, "the priesthood of all believers." So who did the teaching? Any male adherent who demonstrated the ability to avoid consistently embarrassing himself through expounding an unacceptable theological line. This seemed to leave women out of the "all believers" but the inconsistency was never an issue.

The final service of the day involved these self-styled theologians embracing the improbable task of evangelizing the world from the pulpit, a lectern that stood in modest simplicity under the Scripture written in black and gold calligraphy: "Remember Now Thy Creator In The Days Of Thy Youth—Eccl 12:1." What ad hoc committee concluded that, from the entire canon of Scripture, this should be our defining text? And why was the balance of the sentence—"while the evil days come not, nor the years draw nigh, when thou shalt say, I have no pleasure in them"—omitted? Because of lack of space or fear that the subtle warning implied by the completed text would darken the encouraging tone of the opening phrase? We will never know; but every Sunday night one of the men in the assembly, a circuit preacher based in one of the local fellowships, or a visiting missionary rose to the pulpit beneath the gilded text to expound the gospel, each in his own unique way. Rarely did a pagan enter this rarefied atmosphere although perhaps the as-yet-uncommitted youths of the assembly qualified as such, giving practical effect to the sermons and the ecclesiastical banner.

My father prayed publicly at church, either in those basement prayer circles or from the pulpit on rare occasions when he "chaired" the "Sunday night gospel meeting." And my mother sang the occasional solo piece at the same venue. Father handled his responsibilities with some composure but Mother allowed her nerves to interfere with the flow of her adequate voice. In her case the assignment was an aberration of the "women should be silent in the church" theology. I'm not sure how it all fit together but these were significant events for me and as I continue to develop an understanding of the roots of my own prayer life, I see these individual acts of worship as encouragements to be open in my communications with God.

Spiritual Inquisitiveness and Adolescent Sexuality

Somehow the Bible stories and their zealous interpreters combined to draw me into a meaningful relationship with the central figure of Scripture, Jesus of Nazareth. Later, in my teens and early twenties, the occasional prodding by some inspirational teacher would send me into short spurts of theological inquisitiveness. But in spite of the randomness of my biblical research, a theological foundation was established that caused me to seek the narrow way. Somewhere in the vacuum of my adolescent comprehensions came the understanding that there was a true moral road and that Jesus offers an appealing, though often mysterious, approach to the paradoxes of life: "Enter through the narrow gate. For wide is the gate and broad is the road that leads to destruction, and many enter through it. But small is the gate and narrow the road that leads to life, and only a few find it" (Matt 7:13–14).

The options of the narrow and broad roads were evident to me in the confines of my adolescent sexuality. Admittedly these were simpler times. When I earned the right to kiss Doreen D. at Sergie's thirteenth birthday party, Elvis' hips were barely out of diapers. Hugh Hefner hadn't figured out how to make promiscuity and nakedness acceptable on the newsstands. And the so-called "sexual revolution" was a decade away. But hormones are hormones and the '50s were no different from any previous decade or century where people chose to follow their nose or follow a code. I chose to follow a code, a code derived somewhere in the scriptural base I have just described. It is the counter-cultural code of sex only in the context of total commitment. It is part of the narrow way and for some reason I followed it through courtship, engagement, marriage vows, and life. It would be a completely different and extensive essay to describe the consequences of the broad way that is the preoccupation of popular culture and conduct today. The narrow road says conjugation is commitment until death: one flesh. Life can apply stress and strain but only death can tear it apart.

As I eased into and out of adolescence I was surrounded

by peers and elders who drew me into study and prayer in the context of summer camps and small group studies. My world was broadened and although in my early twenties I felt unsure of myself outside of the confines of the church community, my professional life was forcing me out of my cocoon. My marriage to Barb at the age of 25 gave me wings.

Wing to Wing

Twenty-eight years of marriage and four children raised to relative maturity is great cause for praise and I do it now. But prayer within it is a foggy memory. It was just life lived and struggled and prayed in a flash. I can understand why Simone Weil could say, after years of growing in faith and in the middle of writing profound theological insights, "Until last September I had never once prayed in all my life, at least not in the literal sense of the word." I can't quite say that, but while I have a very real sense of God's presence in my life, it seems that the prayers of that period were groanings, yearnings and praise with words hardly uttered. Articulate prayers were utterances formed to fit specific situations rather than genuine outpourings of emotion.

The 28 years referred to above ended in 1994 with Barb's death from cancer. Prayer was often an item of tension between us. Prayer at meal times was quick and shallow, done because of custom. In our rare attempts to pray together I always felt uncomfortable with her "style." That was rather shallow of me. Her prayers were, in fact, a reflection of her expansive love for people, neighbours, friends, family and the strays that fell our way. I now regret that I didn't pursue prayer with her because we could have learned together. We stalled at the point of my misgivings over style but never dealt with that tension other than to fall back to preoccupation with the pressures of our lives.

In the late '80s we attended a couple of John Wimber conferences. This brought us to the point of discussion but, with the emphasis on healing and spiritual gifts, the terms of reference were pretty narrow and didn't deal with the personal issues of praying in the centre of our lives. We tried together to involve ourselves in the Wimber system but a system it was, and neither of us could buy into it, although the worship was new and exciting.

Ironically, it has transpired that both of us have been dealt terminal illnesses. I avoided praying for healing for Barb and, while I do for myself occasionally, it is without any conviction that God has any interest concerning my illness other than making it of use to me in some positive way. So most of my prayers are to that effect.

My conservative upbringing instilled in me an element of stoicism mixed with a theological position: God is finished with all miracles except spiritual ones. By that I mean the miracle of new life through the Spirit. I'm not sure how to deal with such Scriptures as James 5:13–18 which says in part that "believing prayer will save the sick man" (J.B. Phillips) but I believe the Spirit tells me that Scriptures which traditionally are used to support supernatural physical healing have more to do with saving the soul than saving the body. Wimber argued for the power of prayer, suggesting that if we could perfect the system we would eventually raise someone from the dead. I thought, "For what purpose—so they could die a bit later and endure more pain in the meantime? Why would God be concerned about giving someone a little extra toil here when eternity awaits him with a new body?"

It is not that I do not long to stay here. But some days I have had my fill and I live with the tension that Henri Nouwen felt as he lay in a hospital bed, injured from an auto accident but recovering after being near death: this is a bit of a pain. I'm going back to face more of this world.

This sense of resolution about life and death has no doubt been solidified by my experiences in recent years, commencing with Barb's diagnosis of cancer in 1992. I left it to others to initiate prayer for her because my faith was so weak. I don't even recall much resistance on my part in the form of internal anguish before God. Certainly I never really complained to God about it. Barb and I talked about our family but never about our hope. It might have been better if we had, but I don't think it was necessary. We both knew. I told my pastor the wrong person was lying there.

She wrote letters to each child but she never wrote anything to me. And she didn't really communicate a lot to me as her time here wound down. That was due, in part at least, to our inability to discuss issues of faith without running into communication difficulties. I love to throw out wild ideas and debate points of principle. She saw no need to go too deeply into an issue unless it dealt with a practical need. So we held a lifelong truce with the occasional one-sided debate ending in 24 hours of silence. Barb looked after the people; I paid the bills and thought lofty thoughts. It was a passable arrangement.

Cords: Stretched and Broken

With my first "until death do us part" contract fulfilled, it would be almost two years of blissful ignorance before I encountered the numbing reality of my own mortality. Certainly, in retrospect, there were occasions where a physical deficiency puzzled me. As early as the summer of 1993 I found that I was unable to pull myself out of the water when I made my bi-annual attempt at water skiing. In February of 1994 I recall attempting to skip a rock on an icy pond and wondered why the rock took such feeble flight. But it wasn't until the fall of 1995 that I noticed a wasting of the muscle at the base of my thumb, which my doctor diagnosed as carpal tunnel syndrome. This was the only practical defect in my physical life, a difficulty in pressing the space bar on my computer keyboard with my right thumb. I wasted twenty bucks on a wrist brace, little knowing that the support I would ultimately need was a much more complex device. She was waiting for me several thousand miles away and a year and a half down the road. But that's getting ahead of my story.

Oblivious to the neurological train-wreck taking place in my system I began adjusting to the new realities of life. Friends jumped in to fill a few of the empty spots. My partner in business invited me along on their holiday in Hawaii in late August and as a result of my involvement in the Hospice Society, connected with the hospital where Barb died, I had agreed to attend a Hospice and Palliative Care conference in Montreal in mid-September. With a view to diverting our attention from our loss my extended family arranged to spend Christmas in San Diego. Life moved inexorably ahead with its unlimited supply of challenges, frustrations, diversions and minor accomplishments.

Although I was left with a sixteen-year-old son, Fraser, and a twenty-year-old daughter, Karen, still living at home, it was as if I had been released from any direct responsibility to carry on family life as I had known it. In reality such an existence was not possible without the binding warmth of

Barb's personality and gift of hospitality. In addition to my own two children living in the house we had a boarder, a friend of Karen's, and my vain attempts at organizing the workload among us became more of an object of derision than of practical design. Everyone in the household had their own car and consequently went their own way. The house we had lived in for 25 years was the product of endless renovation projects that began even before we owned it. My parents had bought the house in 1961 and had carried out major changes to its original architecture before we bought it from them in 1974. As our family grew we multiplied the sin of attempting to make a mansion out of a molehill. Over time general maintenance took second place to expansion and utility. Bluntly, the place was a mess.

The house was only one of the stretched cords in the fabric of my life. Work was a trial. For years my enthusiasm for my profession as a public accountant had been eroding. I was losing my grip even before Barb became ill. Now it seemed irrelevant since I no longer needed to maintain the lifestyle of the urban neighbour. The options I felt I needed to explore were now completely open to me. But still I hesitated. The fences were down, the field was clear, but there was no definable road.

From Loneliness to Solitude

A few months before Barb's death I discovered, in a used bookstore in Port Townsend, Washington, a copy of a book titled *Reaching Out* by Henri J. Nouwen. It spoke of the three movements of the spiritual life, the first of which he called "From Loneliness to Solitude." Nouwen's second movement of the spiritual life was "From Hostility to Hospitality" describing in detail the godly qualities that typified Barb's life. Somehow the juxtaposition of one essay addressing my imminent need and another describing the person I was about to lose was like a seed drill depositing its cargo in the soil of my anxiety. Something new and rich could grow from the humus of my existence. Faced with the imminent loss of my hospitality partner it intrigued me that the proper end of loneliness could be solitude. The message of the book was one thing, but the "accidental" discovery in such an unlikely place was equally significant. I viewed it as a supernatural event and even as it disturbed my theological conservatism, it introduced a harmonic balance between my experience and my spiritual perspective. And it set in place a hunger for more of the same.

And so it was that in the early stages of my bereavement I was already equipped with the desire to dig deeper into my spiritual roots—to seek out those who would help me move from loneliness to solitude. It wasn't until after that frantic flurry of activity in the fall of 1994, at a wedding in February of 1995, that Dr. James Houston, Professor of Spiritual Theology at Regent College and casual acquaintance of many years, caused me to examine seriously the wide range of options that were available to me. In answer to his question of where I thought my life was now headed, I launched into a litany of my angst over job and vocation, suggesting, facetiously, that maybe I should dump the whole thing and start over. He recognized a man clearly losing track of reality and offered to meet with me. I had no idea where he would lead me or what was motivating him to take time from his Regent College schedule to tutor this distraught basket case—but I said yes. In two short sessions, one over lunch at a local restaurant, and another over dinner at his home, he was able to draw from me some very emotional responses not only to the death of my wife but also to the loss of my father over twenty years earlier. It was as if they were one and the same loss, as if they had left me at the same time. But the quiet caring of this godly man accompanied by a simple meal surrounded by his bulging bookshelves tightened the sagging cords that connected my life to those long-standing spiritual values. I felt secure, surrounded by book-bindings and corralled by brotherly love.

Dr. Houston lent me Jonathan Edwards' *Religious Affections* and gave me a copy of Walter Hilton's *Toward A Perfect Love*, both part of a series titled *Classics of Faith & Devotion*. Both books drew me into the reality of the historical struggle of ordinary people to be faithful to the call of Christ. One section of the Hilton book was particularly significant as it maintains, in the form of two letters to a wealthy convert to Christianity, the need to balance our lives between involvement in vocational pursuits and establishing a spiritual foundation. To these authors I added Thomas Merton, St. Augustine and others as I paddled my way through 1995. The natural result of absorbing the words of these ancient writers was to begin a more diligent and consistent relationship with the source of their wisdom, the Bible: "Your word is a lamp to my feet and a light for my path. I have taken an oath and confirmed it, that I will follow your righteous laws" (Psalms 119:105–6). But there was another inviting path that welcomed me into the two-fold journey of self-discovery and God-discovery.

Looking for Ways to Escape

Parallel to this road of spiritual discovery, I was being drawn into business with my two oldest sons. Kyle had come to a dead end in his personal business endeavour, a company called Ace-In-The-Hole Contracting, an excavation company which was mired in the middle of a lawsuit. He was prevailing upon me to provide capital for a company which would work in the specialized area of concrete formwork. His plan would draw his brother, Craig, who was employed by a company doing similar work, into the fray once we had established our initial contract. Craig was showing special aptitude both in technical carpentry and an application of general construction principles and agreed that he would quit his job when the call came.

Kyle began by throwing a set of drawings on the table indicating the estimated bid would be in the range of $400,000. I suggested we begin by doing a few house foundations but was told somewhat sarcastically that I should get my head out of a place where, once you have it there, it will be very difficult to extract. Somehow I did extract it and in the end we took on several smaller jobs with good profitability and then contracted to build a loft apartment building for a contract price in the area of $200,000, which ended in a lawsuit. Fortunately we had already moved on to more lucrative projects so waiting on the results of our litigation proved to be relatively painless. But pain-free this business was not. To come were ups and downs in financial fortunes which conflicted with the variety of life—changing events that were to parallel them.

Trying a Family Business

The slow but steady growth of our construction company—Whitewater Developments, Ltd.—had blossomed into full-fledged success as we completed a contract involving the redevelopment of a commercial site in West Vancouver during 1996. Our contract was for slightly less than one million dollars and our projected net profit was, after all costs except overhead, in the 25 percent range. During the project every time I prepared the monthly statements I would go to the boys and ask them what they were missing. Thc gross margins were just too good to be true. I was to learn on this project, and thc ones following, that I should never believe the margins we show in the middle of the project. In this case, however, in spite of inflated profits during the course of the project, the end result was still magnificent. But this early success was almost our undoing.

There is no end of opinion on the subject of family businesses. Some will argue that they are recipes for disaster and there is no doubt that when family businesses go the wrong way the fallout among alienated family members is far more devastating than when the participants are simply business associates or friends. You can find new friends but close family members are limited in number and rarely replaceable. While this risk exists it has been my experience that family enterprises can be very rewarding and when an attempt is made to hold to solid business practices the teamwork of family members can create efficiencies not available in arm's-length relationships. Before getting into this tale of undulating fortunes, it would be helpful to describe the varying personalities of its participants.

I have already described the style in which Kyle originally promoted his concept of our commercial venture. From the time he could talk his translation of events was consistently embellished to the point of the listener's disbelief. It was as if he lived in his own bubble with magnified and distorted events taking place within its vicinity. From his earliest days in kindergarten he would provide stories of projects, events or mishaps with hyperbolic verbosity. He could make a minor paint spill sound like a life-threatening disaster. Over time the constant disbelief he engendered created a humorous overtone to the narrative as he slowly backed down from most of the inflated details with a good- humoured smile. Sometimes he would even admit to adding some wild statistic to the story to make it sound better. But there was always an endearing quality about these intense verbal encounters. You could never call him a liar. You would just stand in awe at his "take" on the world and wait for the next amazing event.

This tendency on Kyle's part to expand reality has continued into adult life but somehow it has been turned into creativity. It's as if his view from the bubble makes anything look possible. So it was without a qualm that he launched his first commercial venture, Ace-In-The-Hole Contracting, which he used, in spite of its limited lifespan and dubious success, to launch a construction management career. I would visit him at a high-rise site and be totally mystified as to how this son of mine, this big-talking, fun-loving person, could be given the responsibility of running such a project. But there he was, stomping around with great authority, confidence oozing from every pore. Whatever degree of bravado was involved in Kyle's career development cannot negate the honest hard work applied at each step, beginning as an apprentice in gas fitting and plumbing, working for an excavation company, and finally launching his own enterprise. He had paid his dues.

Craig's journey to this crossroads in our lives followed a less circuitous route. From high school he leaned towards construction trades and immediately began working as a carpenter after graduation. His only financial setback was losing $2,000 in wages when an employer bit the financial dust. After working for a couple of small companies Craig was employed by Micron Construction Limited, one of the largest concrete forming companies in Vancouver. His abilities were recognized quickly and he was given more and more responsibility. Complementing his technical skills was an authoritative but deprecating manner with fellow employees. He told Kyle that when the call came he would jump ship. Sink or swim, he would risk the smaller boat even with Kyle at the rudder.

There is not much to say about my own aptitude for this cause, other than that my capital was required and that my lifelong interest in the physical act of building, partially blinded me to the obvious financial risks. Needless to say my professional accounting experience would fit meaningfully into the management structure. The capital I was providing was hardly equity I could afford to lose. My house was my principal asset but my mental state caused me to throw caution to the wind and I arranged for a $100,000 line of credit against it.

So there are we were, the flamboyant optimist, the freshly trained technician and the risk-taking, frustrated accountant, all ready to fill the empty spaces with concrete. Several years later Kyle was to quip during his toast to the groom at Craig's wedding that "Craig makes all my lies come true." As the accountant I watched the battle on the balance sheet.

A Heady and Dangerous Success

It was Kyle's entrepreneurial zeal which had lured us into this venture and it would be this same quality combined with the blind sheep mentality of his partners that would bring us close to financial disaster, as the heady fumes of success led us into the following year. By the end of our fiscal year, April 30, 1997, we had managed to squander the majority of the capital gained to that point by investing in a number of capital assets including a strata warehouse/ office. During this same period Kyle had developed the keen sense of determination that we should be building high-rises. He had convinced Craig and me that we were ready. I think I was the most guilty since I knew we were not ready, but my preoccupations with other things just let that happen. So we were awarded a contract by Ledcor Industries, Ltd., a giant general contractor, to complete all concrete formwork for a 14 story high-rise in the West End of Vancouver. The contract value of $1,100,000 included several layers of underground parking, a substantial amount of architectural columns and cornices and 12 floors above ground. I kept asking myself how those numbers matched up with the West Van project which involved no underground work and only a three-story building and separate three level parkade.

On June 21, 1997 I wrote the following in my journal:

Well, I'm out of accounting, and just in time. My left hand has deteriorated to single digit keyboarding and my brain doesn't want to think about digits at all. I have just started receiving some disability and spend more and more time on Whitewater but the growth there scares me. They are talking of a payroll of 50 people and we don't really have the capital for that. Kyle has hired a salaried superintendent for the high-rise project with the idea that he would buy into the company but I have had no success in pinning down the potential for this or the timing.

While the new business developed I attempted to motivate myself in my profession with limited success. My mind was increasingly elsewhere. I was drawn on the one side to reading and contemplation. This was countered in the business realm by my greater interest in the hands-on running of our own family company. Further, I was underwhelmed in my lack of interest in promoting the business of public accounting. I was looking for ways to escape. One beautiful spring day the frustrations of my professional struggle drove me from my office to the rocks and beach surrounding the Point Atkinson Light House. My state of mind is reflected in a journal entry from May 3, 1995.

Oh Lord, why am I here on West Beach so low and lost? So far from any help but you!!! What next? What answers lie in these rocks and waters? Or in the lighthouse with no light shining from it—only on it from a source as far away as you seem to be? My voiced prayers fall in the cracks of these rocks as the sounds of helicopters, planes, seagulls and pulsing water respond, but not you. Are you dealing with other things? If I knew what, I would go and try to solve them and then you could tell me what to do next. I thought if I just randomly went somewhere that some amazing thing would happen that maybe it would all fall into place—but nothing like that has taken place here. Only peace—just peace—no answers—just a vacuum and a gentle breeze from the west on my back where the sun lands as well-mixed temperatures that provide a sensual message that maybe peace requires. So is that the amazing thing I look for? Can the normal be amazing? I guess so but it's still no answer. Not for the stuff that still lies waiting for me to return to.

Looking back, I wonder what the fuss was about. What was "waiting for me to return to" was nothing more than the standard struggles for equilibrium in the midst of worldly pressures. Certainly my accounting practice had become a declining economic venture but the construction business with my two sons was, at this point, flourishing. And while the house presented a high-level of anxiety there really was no immediate need for me to do more than eat and sleep there and collect the monthly rental charges from the combination of youthful miscreants that shared the space with me. Maybe my problem was that there were just too many options open to me—too much freedom and not enough discipline. Who can account for why the spirit drops? Possibly the answer is as simple as recognizing that unless it does, we can't experience the rewards of Christ's redeeming power. The miraculous rewards of Jesus' first four beatitudes provide comfort and encouragement to enter into these weaknesses with hope.

"Blessed are the poor in spirit: for theirs is the kingdom of heaven.
Blessed are they that mourn: for they shall be comforted.
Blessed are the meek: for they shall inherit the earth.
Blessed are they which do hunger and thirst after righteousness: for they shall be filled" (Matt 5:3–6).

My Grieving Groping Spirit

True to the promises of Scripture my spiritual senses were being renewed. In my married life I believe I had allowed Barb to lead the spiritual war. She was an evangelist and she lived a life of love and care for friends and neighbours. My heart was with her in full support but my mind was farther afield, straining over career and a couple of failed investments. At times my erratic moods and borderline depression brought her to exasperation. Now I began to regret my doltish behaviour with no way to make restitution other than to reform my own life in some tangible way. Something deep in my grieving, moody, tired but groping spirit told me that this had something to do with digging deeper into the structure of the faith that had led me this far.

My partners in the accounting business were well aware of my state of unrest and had agreed in our February 1995 business review that I should take a three-month sabbatical from the practice during the months of July, August and September. Common wisdom says that in such circumstances you should connect with a friend to formulate a set of goals for the sabbatical and then to help you carry them out. My primary desire was to expand my reading program and to spend time in contemplation and prayer with a view to determining a vocational and spiritual foundation for the rest of my life. My appetite for reading had already been whetted but I needed more direction so I called on my friend, Neil Graham, who had done the sabbatical thing, to provide me with some guidance. From his list of recommendations I selected *Space for God* by Don Postema, a seven-week course to help establish a reflective lifestyle based on biblical principles and supported by both ancient and modern writings and art. My sabbatical itinerary was on its way.

My second goal was to complete a project at Pioneer Pacific, a children's summer camp owned by Inter-Varsity Christian Fellowship, where I was on the maintenance committee. I had agreed to raise funds to rebuild the protective fencing along the shoreline and to supervise its construction. The freedom and quiet solitude I experienced as I drove my pickup truck back and forth from Thetis Island to Vancouver via two separate ferries to carry out this project became a mental model of how I imagined life could be. It was the perfect venue for my meditative ambitions.

Finally, my cousin Stephanie and her husband, Michael, operators of a small Christian study centre in Cyprus, had invited me to visit them if I felt the need for respite. The thought of taking my solitude on a geographical ride began to feel appealing. Other travel interests in Europe included accepting another invitation to visit friends near Frieberg, Germany, and a desire to visit a Christian study centre called Schloss Mittersill in Austria. I had been aware, through my involvement with Inter-Varsity Christian Fellowship, of this fourteenth-century castle which had been converted into a Christian conference and study centre in the '60s. I had spoken with a number of people who had spent time there and currently my business partner, Robert Pasman, was on the board of directors. In addition, I had a casual acquaintance with Carl Armerding, the managing director of the study centre operating within the castle, and his wife, Betsy. This, along with the close email relationship that Betsy maintained with my sister-in-law, Elizabeth, would make it impossible for them to avoid taking some mild responsibility for me should I arrive in a lost and desperate state. With these friendly sites confirmed, scattered as they were from northern Europe to Cyprus, I was ready to venture to my travel agent in order to ransom what was left of my credit.

"I Don't Think I'm the Person You are Looking for"

I still needed to reserve a room at the castle so I called one of two names given to me by Robert. One name was male and the other female. Chauvinism told me that female would be the natural gender for a person receiving reservations, so I placed my call to Lynne Westwood, miscalculating the time difference so that I got her in her room far from the registration desk—which she wasn't responsible for anyway. She said in a voice mixed with fatigue and resignation, "I don't think I'm the person you are looking for." So she told me who to call and how the time difference works; I made my arrangements the following day with a person of the male persuasion. But the female voice responding indifferently to my errant call left me with an unexpected curiosity as to the face and form of the source of this mild rejection.

I say "unexpected" curiosity because I had essentially turned off any motivation to place myself in the perilous path of any potential romance. It would not be an exaggeration to say that I could list twenty eligible women within a local phone call who would be pleasant to spend some time with. A name or two floated to the top of the list on occasions when some of the benefits of married life were particularly missed. I will refrain from revealing what benefits I missed the most or the identity of the individuals I imagined could most adequately compensate my loss. But any time I considered making a move the sheer fright of the rumour machine within my circle of acquaintances drove me back to cover.

Relishing Singleness

As much as I missed my old steady married life I began to relish the freedom of movement that comes with singleness. My sabbatical was taking effect. Somewhere in the recesses of my consciousness was the ongoing issue of my vocational dilemma and the chaos surrounding my domestic establishment. But my mind was on the road, an unknown path with unknown consequences. In late September I boarded a British Airways flight to London, leaving everything behind but my future, a few personal effects and several books.

> *So here I sit "alone" with 200-plus people in an airport waiting room, the flight two hours late, wondering what lies beyond the tunnel. Coming back over the city I can see Lonsdale stretching up the hill, though from 10,000 feet it looks flat like a prairie road. Our house is not visible and is probably unoccupied as Karen is no doubt out on the town. But it causes time to compress when I "see" it from this perspective. It somehow embodies what is real in my life—my children. "Embodies" is not the right word really—that would be sad. It's only a house, but that house held them and protected them for most of their lives (all of their lives for Karen and Fraser) and so it naturally encapsulates a lot of emotion. Maybe the thought of moving out of it*

romanticizes it and viewing, at least its location from here, as I move very quickly away from it, intensifies all that it means as an important element in the establishment of my relationship with its most recent occupants.

My reading on this leg includes a book by Henri Nouwen, the well-known Catholic theologian and spiritual writer, titled The Road to Daybreak. *The following quote sums up some current emotions. "It is hard to believe that God would reveal his divine presence to us in the self-emptying humble way of the man from Nazareth. So much in me seeks influence, power, success, and popularity. But the way of Jesus is the way of powerlessness, and littleness. It does not seem a very appealing way. Yet when I enter into true, deep communion with Jesus I will find that it is the small way that leads to real peace and joy."*

As I read my journal notes from previous days, I am aware that the present is more of that narrow way. I know it to be true but the appeals of the broader road are always before us. I succumb consistently. While travelling light and having modest goals in front of me I recall feeling totally free of the shackles of my responsibilities, anticipating the possibilities of the "deep communion with Jesus" expounded by Nouwen, and expressed in the invitation of Jesus, "Come to me, all you who are weary and burdened, and I will give you rest. Take my yoke upon you and learn from me, for I am gentle and humble in heart, and you will find rest for your souls. For my yoke is easy and my burden is light" (Matt 11:28–30).

Sabbatical—Journey Outward, Journey Inward

My first stop was a small town in the South East corner of Germany. My friends, Hilary and Axel Cole and their son,

Sebastian, live in a small town called Sulzburg near the borders of France and Switzerland. On my final day in Sulzburg I picked up my rental car in Frieberg ready to resume my travels to Mittersill. I had arranged that I would drive Hilary to church on Sunday morning. Axel suggested that he would deliver Hillary's and Sebastian's bicycles to church at the end of the service so they could ride home while I ventured on. It was a fabulously ornate Catholic cathedral completely covered with icons and frescos in gold, pinks and pastel blues. The devotional reflection I felt as I gazed at the twenty-foot-high crucifix, suspended from the left side of the church over the congregation on wires, provided dramatic proof that my spiritual perspectives had shifted somewhat from the conservative confines of Central Park Gospel Hall. I felt an ecumenical rush as I filed, with the legal adherents, to the railing to receive communion. No alarm bells went off and the expression on Jesus' face on the crucifix was as if he were saying to me, "It's okay."

Schloss Mittersill is a Christian retreat and study centre which was established in the 1960s by a group of businessman led by Stacy Woods who was at the time the executive director of an organization called The International Fellowship of Evangelical Students (IFES). The Schloss (German for castle) had operated as a hunting lodge for the rich and famous prior to the Second World War and then was taken over by the Nazis to carry out whatever nefarious schemes fitted their demented minds. Once the war was over and a road had been built from Kitzbuhel to Mittersill, the castle no longer held the appeal of a remote destination so it sat in disuse until the owners decided to dispose of it. The purchase was negotiated on extremely favourable terms, and after some evolution in management and use, the castle settled into its current mode of providing theological study for students from all over the world but with special emphasis on attracting Eastern Bloc students through scholarships. It also provides the opportunity for conferences and retreats and for young adults from all over the world to work and learn together as short-term castle staff.

The study centre element of the Schloss Mittersill operation was directed by Carl Armerding. It was he and his wife, Betsy, whose hospitality I planned to tap as I arrived on the heels of my first week of international travel. Of course it would be a lie to suggest that the physical identification of my reluctant registrar was not also somewhat on my mind as I drove through the Alps towards the castle, but I was totally unsuspecting of the effect that this casual meeting would have upon my life.

The Perilous Path of Romance

Starting a new page in my journal is convenient because I may well want to rip it out and burn it later. Shortly after checking into the Schloss on Monday I heard some animated conversation in the courtyard and then looked down to see Carl and Betsy talking to someone whom I assumed could be Lynne Westwood. Yesterday she introduced herself at lunch and we talked a bit. Carl had offered to take me up one of the mountain valleys for some sightseeing and a hike in the afternoon and somewhere in the conversation he mentioned that Lynne was having a private (two person) birthday dinner for Betsy that evening in her flat and that we were invited for an after-dinner chat. So after dinner Carl grabbed a bottle of white wine from the refrigerator and we headed up with the libation, four wine glasses, and some chocolates I had brought for Carl and Betsy. It was a very pleasant evening with much of the talk centred on our "religious" backgrounds. We took side trips to talk about Augustine, one of my current interests, Carl's trips to Eastern Europe and information about family members.

Dreams in the Night

That night I dreamt that Barb had come back. I had only dreamt of Barb once before, and it was on the occasion of a fleeting connection with some sexual tension. This dream seemed long and intense as I tried to explain to Barb that we couldn't marry again as a whole year had gone by and life had just changed. It was as agonizing as I'm sure it would be if your long-lost love came back after you had married someone else.

The next night I dreamt, it seemed, all night of Lynne. But who can fathom or measure dreams? Though, in this case, it lasted the whole night because I couldn't get her off my mind as I fell asleep and then through the night I woke several times knowing I had been dreaming about her. I awoke fully at 3:30 a.m. and called Craig and the kids at my sisters' home where there was a birthday party going on for Craig. But the same preoccupation and dreaming continued for the second half of the night. I woke at 6:00 a.m., had a bath and headed to a quiet spot in the garden to read, write and pray.

In struggling with the issue of remarriage I desired the will of God. From the time immediately following Barb's death I had considered celibacy as a clear possibility while at the same time desiring a marriage relationship. That desire had been intellectual, not emotional. I had no real desire to "search" for "the right one." I believe my attitude (and I have stated this to friends when they offered material suggestions) is that I am not looking—she will just have to show up.

Herein lies the problem posed by meeting Lynne. Has she shown up? And does God really direct these things? Or are we left to choices based on the desires of our hearts or the quivering of our loins?

"Trust in the LORD with all your heart and lean not on your own understanding; in all your ways acknowledge him, and he will make your paths straight" (Prov 3:6–7). What does this proverb, tucked away in the recesses of my mind for years, tell me? First, I'm grateful that this text has been hiding there because I believe its presence has helped me stay on the narrow path. It speaks of trust and acknowledgement that there is an understanding other than my own. It doesn't take away my will and the process whereby I choose a path. Rather as I acknowledge him, and his understanding—principally in Scripture—my path will, at least, be straight.

So what was supposed to be a quiet retreat in the mountains of Austria had turned into an emotional mine field. My protestations that God stays out of the way in planning our lives seemed at risk. How do I explain the coincidence of my first dream—about Barb—at that point when the seeds of a romantic relationship were in hand but not yet planted?

Researching My Infatuation

During our Tuesday evening wine time the initial physical attraction that I felt for Lynne was supplemented by admiration for her which I felt when she shared her spiritual journey. We shared a common interest in Henri Nouwen. Further, I began to understand the simple life of faith she lived by depending on God for all her needs. Not insignificant was the realization of our mutual identity with the Inter-Varsity Christian Fellowship family, which provided a grounding of spiritual and emotional compatibility. Finally, the pleasant ambiance of the four of us in her quaint and medieval Schloss loft apartment with the balcony overlooking the village of Mittersill was the material fuel for my infatuation—and infatuation it was. So we drank the wine and I went home to dream.

It was not just dreams at night. She became my preoccupation during the day. As I cycled, pushing my unconditioned body to its limit, heart pounding, legs protesting, up the hills of the Hollersbachtal, she was always on my mind. A silly concern kept surfacing—that I could die of a heart attack and no one would ever know how my desperate journal entry could have ended. So, I resolved, I would try to end any speculation, hopefully while I still have my health; maybe even before the end of this trip. My mental, spiritual and emotional batteries were mixing up the signals. I prayed that God would help me untangle the wires.

I had already asked Betsy and Carl to go out for dinner with me for the renowned pepper steak at a local restaurant. On the afterglow of our Tuesday evening tipple it seemed logical that Lynne be added to the guest list even though the dinner idea came partly from Betsy's request to have some time to get news from home, including some insights from me about the events in my life, which indirectly had brought me to see them. But I wanted to discover more about Lynne and my feelings for her, so I decided to delay my talk with Betsy and Carl and invite her. Since I had driven down to their apartment to check on dinnertime and arrangements following my bike trip, I asked Betsy to call Lynne at the Schloss and invite her. She did, and Lynne accepted saying that if Brian had some shillings he needs to get rid of, she would be happy to help. Dinner was great and I simply enjoyed all the company and can't, at this point, distinguish the conversation from the night before.

After dinner Betsy and I had our talk. When I recounted

to her the events of the past two years I found myself impetuously unloading the pitiful details of my dreams and preoccupations. Her comments included:

"Lynne is an absolutely beautiful person."

"I have always felt that the right person for Lynne would be a widower—not a 43-year-old unmarried person with no marriage or child-rearing experience."

"Lynne desires a relationship but not someone who will be changing any of her goals or standards to accommodate that."

And a final spiritual directive:

"When thoughts, issues, and emotions are in conflict I offer them up to God."

In summary, her only advice was to see the events of these two days as guideposts to the answer that God has for me. So God does get in the act!

The question of how my life should turn with respect to marriage or singleness was not one I came on this trip to settle. Of course, since I made no indications of amorous intent to Lynne and assuming that Betsy keeps her own counsel on these intimate discussions, I can just slide back out into my known universe and pretend this new complication to my already burdened psyche never happened. After a few days of reflection I can phone Betsy and tell her the guideposts were, instead, fence posts supporting barbed wire.

But my final night brought no relief. The nocturnal preoccupation continued. When I awoke at 3:00 a.m. I found it impossible to get back to sleep. So I attempted to follow Betsy's final directive. God may have been there somewhere receiving my angst and feeding back cosmic intelligence but the wires on my end seemed disconnected. Besides, I still needed sleep. So I got up and took two Tylenol tablets trusting this artificial stimulant wouldn't permanently interfere with my search for greater spiritual understanding.

To Cyprus in Love

My flight arrangements with British Airways were set up in such a way that for a single airfare you could take three excursions from London to anywhere in Europe. So it required that I fly to Cyprus via London. My flight left Munich at 2:00 p.m. so I needed to pack, eat breakfast and be on my way by 10:00 a.m. Lynne was nowhere in sight as I said my goodbyes to Carl and Betsy. As I drove down the driveway, however, she was walking up with a rolling pin under her arm. Hoping her baker's utensil wasn't in hand to fend me off, I stopped to say goodbye and she handed me a package containing Ferreros & JuJubes. My offering to her had been to leave my spare shillings with Betsy to hand on to Lynne. I informed her of this generous gesture, amounting to about $10 Canadian, which was hardly enough to significantly expand her economic fortunes but enough to let her know that at least she was the first person I thought of as I sought to reduce the weight in my change pocket. So I left with the sense that nothing more than the slightest suggestion that the pieces of a simple friendship could be picked up and incorporated into a larger picture. Did either of us detect a flame in the other's eye? We were not to know until later.

The longest and most anticipated part of my trip was to be Cyprus.

My cousin Stephanie and her husband, Michael, had established a residential retreat and study centre in a small village called Drouseia high on the hillside above the southwest coast of Cyprus. Both Michael and Stephanie have varied backgrounds living and working in Israel and the Middle East. Their objective in establishing this facility was to provide respite and training for Christian workers within the eastern Mediterranean. The house and additional buildings were rehabilitated from an ancient goat farm. As I traveled west from Larnica heading for Paphos, my meeting point with Michael, I was probably following the route that Paul and Barnabas took on Paul's first missionary journey. I was hardly on what could be called a Christian pilgrimage but the sense of touching the geographical context of Scripture gave me a moderate spiritual buzz.

> *"The two of them, [Paul and Barnabas] sent on their way by the Holy Spirit, went down to Seleucia and sailed from there to Cyprus. When they arrived at Salamis, they proclaimed the word of God in the Jewish synagogues. John was with them as their helper. They traveled through the whole island until they came to Paphos. There they met a Jewish sorcerer and false prophet named Bar-Jesus, who was an attendant of the proconsul, Sergius Paulus. The proconsul, an intelligent man, sent for Barnabas and Saul because he wanted to hear the word of God. But Elymas the sorcerer (for that is what his name means) opposed them and tried to turn the proconsul from the faith. Then Saul, who was also called Paul, filled with the Holy Spirit, looked straight at Elymas and said, 'You are a child of the devil and an enemy of everything that is right! You are full of all kinds of deceit and trickery. Will you never stop perverting the right ways of the Lord? Now the hand of the Lord is against you. You are going to be blind, and for a time you will be unable to see the light*

of the sun.' Immediately mist and darkness came over him, and he groped about, seeking someone to lead him by the hand. When the proconsul saw what had happened, he believed, for he was amazed at the teaching about the Lord" (Acts 13:4–12).

No doubt I got to Paphos quicker than Paul and Barnabas. An hour and a half by mini-bus to Limassol and an equal leg in a stretched Mercedes taxicab to Paphos and I found myself languishing in a sidewalk cafe with a KEO (one of only two available brands of Cypriot beer—the other Carlsberg) and a tomato sandwich, pondering a way through the Cypriot telephone system, then throwing unfamiliar sequences of numbers at operators who spoke English reluctantly or not at all. Eventually I accessed Michael's telephone answering machine to let him know I had arrived. So I aimed my chair at the taxicab depot across the street, where we had agreed to rendezvous, to wait for his familiar rotundity and white beard to appear.

My difficulties with the telephone system were in spite of Lynne's clear instructions on how to use the prefixes. This bit of assistance, although compromised by my lack of aptitude in following directions, came out of the fact that she had vacationed in Cyprus on a number of occasions visiting friends (author Joyce Huggett and her husband David) who live within a ten-minute drive from Michael and Stephanie's retreat centre. This connection had obviously supplied some grease to the conversational axle at Mittersill. Of course this was one more reason for my mind to continually bend itself in her direction. So as I sat with my beer and sandwich preoccupied with thoughts of her I wrote in my journal (September 29, 1995):

I have written a pile of letters in my mind and vacillate between the bold and the benign. The bold lays it all out and awaits the answer. The benign just begins correspondence without any reference to personal feelings. How could I have said "this is actually fun"? I thought I took this trip to get respite from my complications. Now I'm allowing myself to be drawn into this vortex. It must be love because it feels like a sickness. What the heck is going on? I'm imagining our getting married and I don't even know her. Why is this happening to me?

A Low-risk Inquiry

On the letter writing issue I finally agreed on the benign. At that stage it seemed the safer route:

September 30, 1995—Paphos, Cyprus

Dear Lynne,

As the JuJube population diminishes in my beautiful room at Drouseia , thoughts of you and the Schloss continue to delay shifting my entire being into this new experience. So I have just read all the material I took away to torture myself for not arranging to stay a little longer at Mittersill.

The apple snack was right on the money, supplemented by airline cheese that I got on my flight from Frankfurt. And what more can we say about Ferreros & JuJubes? So thank you for your thoughtfulness. And the Cyprus map was a comforting presence as I attempted to contact Michael from a phone booth in Paphos—where I was using one too many digits in the number and getting nowhere with various telephone company operators.

The taxi trip here was all you implied it might be. A Cyprus taxi is a good place to re-confirm that you are completely in God's hands. He decided to keep me here for another day.

Once Michael and I made contact he took me on a varied tour including his own errands, a visit to a Greek coffee shop operated by a couple and their daughter who are Greek refugees from the 1974 Turkish invasion—and a variety of ruins, both Roman and Turkish, accompanied by a mass of historical facts. We got "home" by 7:00 p.m. and then out for suckling pig at a local restaurant. There's my life between then and now.

One very pleasant stop on our tour was Jerusalem House, a hospice in Paphos where Michael and Stephanie are involved as volunteers. There is only one patient, a 92-year-old lady named Rosina whom they "rescued" from Larnaca where she was receiving no attention. Having an active interest in hospice and palliative care for a number of the years in North Vancouver, arising in part because of my experience with my wife, it was extremely comforting to find myself in these quiet surroundings and to be able to comfort someone so estranged from the normal functions of life. I have plugged into the 24-hour care cycle and will be going back for a two-hour shift tomorrow. I hope to get a photo of her and give it to the hospice to place somewhere honouring their first resident.

Today I spent the afternoon fixing the kitchen sink in the house here so considering how much time I have spent working on my own house during my sabbatical I guess this qualifies as the "busman's holiday."

I have been praying for you and for confirmation in your next steps in vocation and mission. Betsy reminded me of the concept of patiently waiting for the "guideposts" as I struggle with some of the same issues. Some have already appeared by the side of my road and I trust the same is happening for you.

Please count on my support in prayer and finances for whatever path you follow.

Sincerely,
Brian

This travelogue style letter seemed a safe response to our brief meeting and final gift exchange. The slight shift at the end to some personal comments about my involvement in the hospice movement might even win me some humanities points. No harm in promoting your sensitive side in matters of the heart. The letter was composed over the time I spent in Cyprus but wasn't posted until I arrived in England, several days later.

Re-entry

A surprising last minute upgrade to business class on my British Air return flight provided a deceptively smooth descent back into the complexities of everyday life. My three-month sabbatical was over but the seeds of change had been fertilized by my spiritual and geographical travels. The initial success of our construction company contrasted dramatically with the continuing sense of personal frustration with and the lack of growth in my accounting practice. One huge blow was the loss of significant revenue from a major client because of the sale of his principal business.

Even though I had arranged with my sons for discounted accounting charges to Whitewater, our family company had become my largest client.

Reflecting on my career in public accounting I could say that I enjoyed the science of it but never the business. It seems that whenever there was an opportunity to use my accounting knowledge to involve myself in business other than accounting I would drift off in that direction. It had happened in the ill-fated real estate venture in which I was a principal participant during the '80s. Once again it was happening. In the end these proved to be distractions from my regular professional work. But now, when reviewed in context, these experiences support my sense that, if I'd had the courage, I would have jumped ship years ago. The right time and the courage were meeting and shaking hands.

So here I was back in the land of endless possibilities but with one new ingredient to stir the fog of confusion, a woman lodged thousands of miles away—a woman who was no more aware of my feelings for her than she was of the state of my mind. But none of this changed the reality that two businesses needed my attention and the daily quota of decisions had to be made. Any course of action that involved divesting myself of an accounting practice would take time and, despite my predilection towards making the move, I felt frozen in combat.

With Care and Trepidation

Not long after my return I received a short note from Lynne. Although it made no reference to any of the subjects I dealt with in my letter to her, for some reason I assumed it was a response. This, in spite of the fact that she asked questions about Cyprus—which, to some degree, I had addressed. Somehow I had neglected to realize that my paltry gift of leftover shillings provided a reason for her to write on her own. Regardless of my inability to sort out that simple question I happily read and re-read the letter trying to determine its level of cordiality. Only my lack of personal confidence kept me from concluding the obvious but even I, in my fragile state, saw reason to be optimistic. She was on the same train.

October 15, 1995—Mittersill

Dear Brian,

It's Sunday afternoon. I'm sitting in the sun on the balcony. We've had two weeks of magnificent weather. Bright blue sky, lush green meadows, the trees a mix of brown, green, yellow, orange but alas no red! We gaze at the beauty and praise God. I wish you could see it here today. It's really extraordinary.

I've been wondering how your time in Cyprus was. Did you find the beach? Enjoy some Greek food? Greek wine? Greek beer? I'm so sorry that the Huggetts weren't there—today David Huggett spoke about transition, leaving what is good—being in what seems like a desert—but then allowing God to prepare us, show us new things, readying us for the next stage. You would enjoy David.

For me Cyprus has been a wonderful and a hard place. It's been a lonely place but also a place where I've experienced my loneliness moving to solitude, about which Nouwen speaks. So, I'm excited about my two weeks in January in Cyprus and also a little nervous. Joyce Huggett tells me that she thinks I should holiday for a week and then she'll "put me into silence" on retreat for a week. A week of silence for me can be a bit of a challenge (smile).

The Board meetings were quite stressful for me. I'm feeling quite affirmed by people but stressed by the decision I must make. I don't want to sound too pious but I really want to be in the centre of God's will. It might not be the easiest place, but it is the only place to be. I just wish he'd send a telegram telling me where that is!

It was good to meet you here. Thanks for dinner and lunch. Come back soon!

With care,
Lynne

Emboldened with the phrases "Come back soon!" and "with care, Lynne" ringing in my head, I carefully composed and posted my second letter in which I blew the code:

October 26, 1995

Dear Lynne,

Though I can't match the tranquil time and setting you describe for your letter writing, the view out my office window at 8:30 a.m. this Thursday morning needs also to be credited to God's generosity, if for no other reason than that he has given me the "red" you long for, so I can describe it to you. A variety of deciduous trees front the building across the street and the sun is bathing them with muted morning light in a variety of shades of red....

Cyprus. Too much to cover in this letter but in answer to your direct questions: 1) Did you find the beach?—No!; 2, 3 & 4) Enjoy some Greek food? Greek wine? Greek beer?—Yes! Also some Greek brandy. The wine is expensive, to say the least, and quite good; the beer very political (you probably know that Carlsberg is right-wing and KEO is left) so you vote every time you buy; and the food, dominated by "kleptico" in my experience, was excellent.

My best food experience was at a classy restaurant in the town on the coast, the name of which I can't remember. But the most interesting was at a Greek wedding reception in a roadside taverna where, along with about 500 guests seated in multiple rows of tables, we had pork kleptico, Carlsberg and wine followed by a major "money pinning" ritual as family and guests took turns draping the bride and groom with Cypus monetary notes of various denominations. Michael Wood says they usually receive in excess of 10,000 pounds... sometimes up to 30,000. This seems like a pretty exciting way to start married life though this particular pair didn't show it. A striking element of the affair was the sad and vacant look of the bridal couple, almost matched by the sombre composure of most of the guests....

I suppose it's time to broach the obvious point that this letter is not being written simply to answer your questions about Cyprus. My contact with you at the Schloss has caused rumblings in my central nervous system (I suppose that could also be referred to as "heart") that have not been easy to ignore. I have analyzed your letter continuously since its arrival looking for evidence that another letter from me might be welcomed and trust that my conclusion, which has encouraged this bold paragraph, was correct.

My life since my wife's passing has been blessed by so many things: the encouragement of my children and friends; the help of one friend in particular in dealing with the grieving process; a real and meaningful search for the personal God who wants a deeper commitment from me; and with and around those issues a desire to know, as you expressed it yourself, the will of God in my life. Insofar as that relates to our correspondence you must understand I have no objective other than to at least feel his will in it and your response will be taken as an additional sign of that, not the reverse. But considering the nature of our individual positions in life, including geographically, I think the acknowledgement of emotions is best expressed sooner than later. Does that sound terribly verbose? (These two paragraphs have been written ten times in my mind, some of the versions probably worded better than I have managed here, but this will have to do.)

The last thing I want for you is more trauma or confusion. But the relief for me from emoting is immense even though the dropping of this letter into the irretrievable blackness of a mailbox will be akin to the launching of a small boat into river rapids. I may sink; I may have a great ride; but I won't get the boat back on shore until I'm down the stream a bit. But don't be afraid to sink me. I have a number of flotation devices.

If I knew you were going to Cyprus I had forgotten but would like nothing better than for you to show me "the beach" in person and to talk about solitude and Henri Nouwen.

I have disguised this letter somewhat in a Pasman Smith envelope in case a second personal letter from me filtering its way through your front office causes unwanted rumours (and related stress). If further correspondence is encouraged in your response you can also tell me what form and route that might take.

The terribly business-like style of this letter is a result of its being written at my office computer when I should be cranking out chargeable time but it might have been tougher to write if I couldn't be somewhat cerebral.

With care and trepidation,
Brian

Any rational person would have concluded, based on the tone and texture of Lynne's letter to me, that she was going to be receptive to my literary advances. But I was still in a state of shock as to the depth of my own feelings after such a casual encounter and couldn't comprehend reciprocation. So, somewhat blinded by my own insecurity, I began to doubt the bold representation I had made in my letter the instant it left my hand. Added to my anxiety was the sheer uncertainty of advancing so suddenly into a relationship which, I thought, would only add to the complexities of my life. As time progressed I would discover exactly the opposite.

Ominously Hopeful Symptoms

Possibly as early as 1994 I had noticed a slight wasting of the muscle at the base of my right thumb. It was becoming difficult even to press the space bar on my computer. I experimented with an ergonomic keyboard but that had a greater tendency to paralyse my mind than relieve my thumb, so it was soon abandoned. When I took the time to consider this minor disability it brought surges of anxiety. What could be causing this and what kind of treatment could possibly correct it? Finally, on my return from Cyprus, I visited my doctor. His diagnosis of carpal tunnel syndrome resulted in a treatment (a brace for my right hand). But there was no relief for the occasional anxiety. I was skeptical of his "let's take a shot at this one" diagnosis.

Should it be surprising that I would decide at this point to succumb to the lure of the libido factory, the local fitness gym? My friend Randy, evangelistic body builder extraordinaire and sales rep for Empire Fitness World, sold me on the idea that for an annual fee of $269, discipline and a substantial amount of physical effort I could become a trim, coping member of society. I don't doubt for a minute that somewhere in my motivational inventory was the idea that I needed a better looking body if I was about to get serious in romance. Somehow my vanity told me that moving ten pounds six to ten inches higher on my torso would advance the cause of love. So I began "working out."

One month after my return from Europe, filled with the frustration of work—having discovered that several doubtful accounts receivable in my accounting practice had moved from the doubtful category to being very unlikely—and still with no firm take on the status of my romantic pursuits, I decided to escape to our summer cabin at Buccaneer Bay, three hours by auto, ferry and motor boat from my home.

Hoping for a Positive Answer

The ferry would come in an hour and I was carrying an unopened letter from Lynne which, I assumed, contained an answer to my current obsession—her. I came home from work to go to Buccaneer Bay with no thought that my letter would be answered this soon. When I saw the letter on the entrance stand I assumed that it must be from Betsy, but there on the corner of the envelope were the initials "L.W."—a hint, though ever so remote, that the answer would be "yes." I had asked her where and how I should write if she wanted me to continue and it seemed the "L.W." was to provide anonymity.

I refrained from opening the letter, partly from fear but mostly because I had weighed the advantage of having a couple more hours to hold the feelings of hope against the possibility of sacrificing the feeling of relief that I might get from a "yes" answer. Or perhaps I was avoiding the despair of a "no." I imagined opening the letter sitting in my boat or on the beach in the fading light. And since I was going to be completely useless for a little while no matter what the answer, I might as well be at the Bay with my mind on the centre of the universe, Jesus, the one on whom my affections must be centred no matter what my fate in love or war.

> *It is November 3, 1995. I was shocked to find on opening my piece of mail in the dark (having set a fire in the fireplace) that the letter was not a reply to my last letter but a reply to my first. Lynne had written to me before she received my first letter. I can fly myself to Europe in a day but it takes an envelope two weeks!*

Anyway, I though I had my answer.

I will spare my embarrassment to the reader by not recounting here the list of clues from the first two letters that I entered in my journal as evidence that Lynne was in the game. It will be sufficient to recount that included with the letter was her personal newsletter directed to her financial supporters and next to an item indicating her intention to take a two-week holiday in Cyprus she had written "Want to come?"

The Heart Soars as the Body Sinks

> *Meanwhile I have been to the fitness club three times this week to do my "Randy" routine. But all this exercise seems to be doing more to my body than build it up. The routine of exercise seems to bring a sense of calmness though I have feelings in my midsection that make me think I have some virus that is eating my nerve endings. My appetite is good and I feel great otherwise, though the "butterflies," tiny nerve twitching feelings that flit about my middle region, continue.*

On November 16, having spent the day at a motivational seminar with my partners, I came home to "the letter" from Lynne. I ran a bath, got into it to soak my sorry butt and legs and opened the letter. Though it has not yet been spoken in so many words I believe it is love we feel for one another. Can it ever be brought to fruition? The bus that is my body seems to be breaking down just as it is coming to a very important station.

The letter was everything and more than I could possibly have hoped for. If it were not for a lot of discomfort in my back and upper left leg area from something I woke up with, combined with the continuing stomach problem, I would be able to revel completely in my good fortune of discovering that our feelings are mutual. But I tried to wipe my silly health concerns out of my mind (I had a doctor's appointment the following day) and arrange some thoughts for my telephone call to Lynne.

> *The doctor examined me about the stomach twitching. He had no light to shine on the situation. But today the twitching feelings seem to be accelerating by the development of back and leg pain when I get out of bed. My mental health, as a result of worry about my physical health, has deteriorated, probably made worse by confirmation from Lynne that she has had, in her words, "a stirring in my heart" since I left.*
>
> *Is this some tragic irony that this happy humbling news comes the very day that some insipid disease takes hold of my body? To have the heart soar when the body sinks is a truly despairing place to be. But there is no question it's where I am. So the joy I feel just in knowing that Lynne's "heart is very warm" toward me is being struck*

down into an abyss of mental pain—pain that just won't go away—and I sense the symptoms themselves in my body are fundamentally incapacitating.

The euphoria of the week had been spoiled by depression and pain. I had tried to hand this over to God but he hadn't taken it.

To find solace I read chapter twelve of Joyce Huggett's, *Encountering God.* The subject is "In Pain." She started with Isaiah 66: 11–12:

"Oh, that you may suck fully of the milk of her comfort,
That you may nurse with delight at her abundant breasts,
As nurslings, you should be carried in her arms and fondled in her lap,
As a mother comforts her child
So will I comfort you."

As I wrote down these words it came upon me. I felt Jesus was and always is with me now. But what kind of a journey was he taking me on?

With our communication frequencies synchronized I made my first phone call to Lynne. Unfortunately my calculation of the time difference between Canada and Austria was not precise, so she found herself adjusting to a sudden shift in communications medium at 2:00 in the morning. After a quick apology I left her to finish her night's sleep, although in fact it was to continue in fitful wonder at whom she had become hooked up with.

Once normal telephone communication lines were firmly established and we settled into the casual recounting of each day's events, it soon became clear that we needed some time together to check the emotional thermometer. I quickly rationalized that another two weeks away from work would make no significant difference to my fragile financial position. So we agreed to meet in Munich in January to fly together to Cyprus. Lynne arranged for separate condominiums in the apartment complex where Joyce Huggett lives and holds spiritual retreats near the oceanfront town of Polis.

In the meantime, I was having quite a time trying to drum up enthusiasm for anything but going to see Lynne. I had an awful time getting going in the morning but that turned out to be a blessing because it sent me back to *Space for God* and other reflective material, including my Bible.

Courting in Cyprus

My seatmate on the flight from London to Munich was an American working for Andersen Consulting in Germany. We swapped love stories over France. He had fallen in love with his dentist. My story was still in the making and when I told him the object of my suspected affections was waiting for me at the Munich airport and that we were heading into the city for the night, he offered to drive us to our destination. Consequently the romantic rendezvous I had sheepishly constructed in my imagination was turned into a formal introduction between my date and my driver. The disappointment of this diversion from my imagined game plan was far outweighed by the convenience of the delivery system. After a short wait near the baggage carousel, feeling somewhat ill at ease for the delay, I finally spied a somewhat familiar looking figure striding towards us. Despite my normal ineptitude, a visual form of dyslexia at recognizing faces, I was able, in this case, to recognize the smile that had so completely disarmed me less than three months before.

Lynne had arranged for us to stay with friends who were in the United States diplomatic corps. So our destination was the American Consulate. Holding hands discreetly in the back seat of a stranger's car, attempting to include its owner in our conversation, we began our journey of physical discovery. After directing us to our rooms to deposit our luggage, Kelly and Bill Graves, our sensitive hosts, allowed us a few quiet moments in their living room to talk and negotiate a quick hug and a kiss while they prepared dinner. Three months of correspondence and telephone conversations made our reunion almost too natural compared with the build-up of anticipation. But the smile that still greets me each morning as she comes to release me from my overnight breathing machine and to begin the daily ritual of raising my languid torso to its fighting position in a power chair, was there in all its glory. My heart was on a sure path and my lips didn't stumble.

Our Lufthansa flight took us directly to Paphos, where we were met by our host, Joyce Huggett. No long Cypriot taxicab ride on this trip; just a short drive to our condos. Joyce introduced us to our respective accommodations, let us know where she could be found, and left us to find our way on this continuing journey into one another's hearts.

We were soon to realize that Mediterranean housing is designed for the eight to nine months of temperate climate that typifies the region. The few months of cool temperatures don't justify central heating or conventionally powered water heating and we had arrived in the middle of winter. Solar water heating works when the sun shines and since it rarely does that at night there was no hot water when you want it the most—first thing in the morning. To counter this shortcoming in the system, there was an electrical auxiliary system that provided a limited amount of hot water within a half-hour of turning on the switch. Each condo also sported a small electric heater, shaped like an old hot water wall unit, with wheels. My morning routine involved a quick scamper over freezing terrazzo, a flick of the hot water switch, a frantic relocation of the electric heater into the bathroom while sliding the electric cord under the door to the hallway socket, and a mad dash back to bed and a half-hour wait for the water to warm and the bathroom atmosphere to mellow.

In fact I knew from my previous visit to Cyprus that we would not be basking in relentless sunshine, but it had not occurred to me that houses made of concrete and terrazzo without central heating could act so effectively as refrigerators once the moderating rays of the sun have disappeared. This initial climatic shock, combined with jet lag and the possible effects of my as yet undetected disease, made the first few days in Cyprus a blur of self-doubt and agitation. At one point I even suggested to Lynne that I cut short my stay to one week. To this day I'm not sure what emotions filled her being when she heard this cop-out proposal. But Lynne's encouragement to soldier on must have been enough to drag me out on various excursions and eventually the days turned into enjoyable routine. One daily event that strangely capped most days and drove us into each other's arms under a warm blanket was the 5:00 p.m. television airing of that vintage American horse opera, "High Chapparal." This corny drama and a Vancouver-based cooking show called "The Urban Peasant" were the only North American television shows airing in Cyprus. Out of this elite selection we chose the former as our afternoon cultural stimulation and often raced home from some other activity to catch it.

Both of us had come to love the town of Paphos. We had both visited the Roman ruins and mosaics that dominate the tourist tracks and had delighted to spend time walking around the tiny harbour, where pelicans chase tourists for handouts, and where every Sunday afternoon the main thoroughfare becomes a small town drag strip where whole families hang out the windows of their cars as they drive up and down taking in the action that they themselves are creating. There were an equal number of large women as men driving the family cars with the children and grandparents jammed in the back seat.

Discerning our Marriageability

Joyce had agreed to meet with us individually so that we could tell our respective stories, express our angst and seek an independent perspective on our fast-track love affair. Joyce and Lynne had been friends for years (my knowledge of Joyce was limited to having read one of her books). Lynne would go and visit Joyce in the morning and I would drop in for an hour in the afternoon. We both looked forward to the more warmly furnished and electrically heated atmosphere of her condo, not to mention the hospitality of her charming counsel and a hot cup of tea. Later in our stay Joyce's husband David returned and we were able to spend time with both of them. In the end, their affirmation and friendship helped us conclude our paths were somewhat parallel.

Our time in Cyprus was coming to an end, but we were in Paphos and we were in love. So we grabbed each other's hand and headed for the beach to watch the sun go down and find a quiet place to eat. We walked again out onto the breakwater to sit in the sun. What is there about a sunset that re-sets the time clock in your head? Everything is now: spread in random colours over the sea and sky like different coloured inks on a blotter. The past was back over my shoulder, in shadows but still visible; the future somewhere in that glowing horizon where the sun was about to go. As I sat there, I felt the seeds of a whole new thing germinating. But somehow the crushing speed of the events that had recently overtaken my life made me ask myself how much harder can it get. Lynne sat beside me bearing her own thoughts. I knew I was going to ask her to step grandly into the muddle of mine.

We headed back into town to find a place to eat and settled on Mother's Restaurant, where a small fire flickered in a central hearth and where its few patrons preferred tables along the wall. Strains of '50s and '60s music filtered through the atmosphere backed up by quiet talking and some dishes rattling in the kitchen. We took a place by the fire, locked our fingers in the middle of the table and smiled at each other. There was a tangible confidence between us that our lives would work well together. The issue of marriage had already been broached on several occasions. There was really only one question. Do we jump now or separate to carry on courting by phone and email and wait for some more blessed time? The waiter arrived, pretending to ignore our preoccupations, and presented us with the menu.

Once the formalities of ordering, serving and small-talking with the waiter were completed (he quickly became known to us as Costas, the owner) and as we were able to introduce ourselves to the lamb and red wine, I said to Lynne, "Will you marry me?"

She paused, smiled, snaked her hand through the table debris to mine and said, "Yes." After spending our time over dinner making plans we asked the owner for a copy of the tape he was playing, told him we would come by for it in a couple of days, and headed home realizing we had missed "High Chapparal."

We returned together to Schloss Mittersill. Lynne now had the answer to the question she posed to herself about my being part of her life after discovering that her first words to me over the phone, "I don't think I'm the person you want" did not reflect reality. After a few short months of correspondence and telephone conversation, and less than three weeks of personal contact, we decidedly wanted each other.

At the earliest convenient time we phoned Lynne's parents in Toronto to tell them the news of our engagement. Suddenly I found myself talking to a man I had never met, a man who was warning me that the person who was about to become my domestic partner had no money and could not cook. I told him I was just going to have to overlook those deficiencies and work with what we had. I didn't have the equivalent family unit to advise, so I decided to wait until I got home to gather my troops and fill them in, face-to-face.

No one seemed particularly surprised by the results of my trip. I suppose the volume of propaganda that I had verbally distributed about this woman made my pilgrimage a mere formality to them. So my life returned to normal. And normal included the health issue. The messages being transmitted through my nerves and muscles held an unmistakably ominous ring, which I had been able to ignore in the exhilaration of travel and courtship. Shortly after my return home I began to chronicle my mental and physical state.

Someone Else will Carry You

On February 5, 1996 I woke at 5:00 a.m. with that persistent stomach uneasiness and in my horizontal state I had a sense of dread surrounding every task I considered. After about 45 minutes in this condition I finally got up to deal with my life again. Fraser was sick and called down to me to bring him some ginger ale. So I went down to the 7/11 to get some. After a breakfast of frosted Mini-Wheats and after having done some kitchen cleanup, I got to my desk at 7:45 a.m. for some spiritual orientation, feeling pretty good, but wishing I could stay home all day and not go out to face it all. I guess I'll have to, I decided.

I couldn't concentrate on my Bible so I spent some time meditating and waiting on God, as the warm currents drifted up from my electric heater under the desk, and the rain drifted down, rain that cleared the snow from my back yard and driveway and caused ripples on my skylight. I prayed for endurance.

The next day I woke again at 5:30 a.m. I began to think that I had to view this as a fundamental change in my system. Start thinking of less sleep and just get up and "do it." I was wimping out thinking about my health, but I was due to see Dr. Ray Penner about my wrist and I thought my concerns about that would spill over into the rest of me.

My brother, Graeme, took me to lunch yesterday and I talked to him about spending some time on my house. I really need to concentrate on Pasman Smith & Co. and let others do the work on the house. But as far as PS & Co. is concerned, I have a growing feeling that I must withdraw from it. As I read "Day Four—Encounter With Christ" of A Seven Day Journey With Thomas Merton *and meditate on its contents, I know that I must put his comment at the top of my "mission" statement: "God calls human persons to union with Himself and with one another in Christ." I think my feelings and anxieties about my role as a public accountant are God's way of telling me my real place is elsewhere. I must make the break.*

Accepting Reality

On April 1 Dr. Makin, the second specialist I had seen, after the first cursory examination, said he needed to see me again for about an hour to conduct some tests. I had said jokingly to Robert Pasman, my business partner, when I left the office for the appointment, that I was going to see if I had ALS. So this idea of more tests supported my sense that this was something more than carpal tunnel syndrome.

My mind is now confirming what my body has been telling me. It is on an accelerated path to the place they all go. It has ALS. That conclusion may be premature because the doctor glibly hands out a 25 percent option of something else, a nerve pinched in the upper spinal column brought on, possibly, by a "benign" cyst. But my body also tells my mind that this is not likely.

Immediately, I started to become oppressed by the multiplying issues in my life: selling the house; planning for two trips away; a wedding in September; concern over Fraser's future with the changes in my life forcing them on him; and continuing frustration over my accounting practice (lack of growth; lack of concentration on my part; difficulty in collecting accounts—even from clients that are loaded); and missing Lynne every minute of the day and wondering how, or if, in my clouded state, I would ever get to my own wedding.

Three days later I went to Dr. Ray Penner and when he asked how I was, I broke into tears. It didn't take him long to diagnose depression and he prescribed Prozac, which I gladly accepted in the hope that it would solve all my problems. While he advised me that it takes a couple of weeks for the drug to take hold, I was still surprised to find myself in a very deep state of anxiety on the following Thursday, the day before I was to see Ray again. I called Mike Nichols, one of my pastors, and he came to talk and pray with me. He advised me not to push myself to work, so I stayed home all that day and the next until I went to my appointment with Ray at 1:15 p.m. feeling much better.

Finally, I had my appointment with Dr. Makin on April 16, and after electric shock and needle tests I was told of my possible fate. We set an appointment for an MRI the next day, after X-rays of my eyes to make sure there were no metal fragments that might come bursting out under the intense magnetic force of the imaging process, the results of which I would discover the following Tuesday, April 23.

I awoke the next morning after a troubled sleep to read the last chapter of the Gospel of John, where Jesus is speaking to Peter challenging him three times about his commitment to him. After Peter answers, "You know that I love you" (v. 17), Jesus says, "Feed my sheep. I tell you the truth, when you were younger you dressed yourself and went where you wanted; but when you are old you will stretch out your hands, and someone else will dress you and lead you where you do not want to go." Then in verse 19 it says, "Jesus said this to indicate the kind of death by which Peter would glorify God." Finally Jesus said to him, "Follow me!"

I want to do both of those things—to glorify God in my death and to follow Jesus—no matter where I am led and what kind of death I experience. I pray continually that God will enable me to do it.

Why Not Me?

Why me? That's the question to ask now, isn't it? It seems strange to realize that I have asked more often, when I observe someone else in deep trouble or questionable health, the question "why not me?" Some will argue that God sends these trials to us for a higher purpose.

Of course, as soon as I was certain of the ALS diagnosis I phoned Lynne to inform her. In a tearful conversation I offered her the option of pulling out. She insisted she had no intention of doing that.

The body-chilling waves that sweep over me on waking make the mornings hard to deal with, and the mornings come early. It seems that each successive morning I wake up a little later. This morning at 3:45 a.m.; yesterday at 3:15; the first morning of this adventure at 1:30. I am able to get some sleep from first waking, but each time I awake again the same realization hits me, and my body reacts to the fear as if a bucket of turpentine had been poured over it. The first time I had that feeling I was sitting in a chair in Dr. Makin's office as he told me my odds.

I wake for good at 6:15 a.m. and got up fifteen minutes later to make another attempt at taking life "a day at a time." I am now reading the Gospel of Luke and in 2:36 I read: "There was a prophetess, Anna, the daughter of Phanuel, of the tribe of Asher. She was very old; she had lived with her husband seven years after her marriage, and then was a widow until she was eighty-four." What does this mean? Hardly anything else has been on my mind except wondering how long I will live and hoping that the grim stages of this illness wouldn't last too long. So is this a promise from God that it won't be more than seven years? I trust it's not a promise that Lynne would never marry again.

The next day I woke early as usual and did some Whitewater work before heading down to the office. Once there, I discussed with both Andrea and Robert separately our decision to advance the wedding date. As well, I expressed my resolve to change my modus operandi through the sale of my part of the practice to my sister, Andrea, and to operate on a purely locum basis doing administration, file work or bookkeeping.

Then I headed south via the Albion ferry to go to clients and friends, Al & Sue's in Langley to deliver tax returns and the bad news of my predicament. Sue was not home yet, and after I said maybe I would just drop off the returns and go,

Al immediately asked me what was wrong. I was somewhat surprised by his insight. Although I thought I was hiding my stress I must have looked like someone trying to find a firm footing. So I said, "Sit down with me and I'll tell you how I'm feeling." Tears came to his eyes and the word "fuck" came from his mouth, simultaneous expressions of sorrow and anger. Then he just got up from his couch, came and sat beside me and put his arm around me and I joined him in a bawl, my first on this issue, and it felt good. Also the camaraderie I felt with this man, who has always treated me fairly and whose affections for certain people shone clearly through his tough business hide, felt good. He left his arm around my neck for a long time as we discussed the fairness issue, one that always seems to come up, as well as our respective understanding of how God fits into the picture.

We had red wine, wonderful barbecued steak, baked potato and a shrimp and avocado salad. I ate less than I normally do, but I still ate too much and drove home with a mixture of not only elation for such a wonderfully warm commiseration but also a sense of dread as I drove into the night alone with the ominous fear of another bad night's sleep.

I wasn't disappointed. It passed all expectations. Torture. For the two and a half hours from 11:30 p.m. to 2:00 a.m. my mind hallucinated, one of those nightmares that just kept recurring every time I slipped out of consciousness, leaving me with the impression that I didn't sleep at all. Most of the time, I was writhing with agitation in my legs and stomach, and perspiring through feet and hands between sheets that had already absorbed too much of the same treatment the three previous nights. Things can only get better, I hoped. Then, after casting aside the idea of phoning Bill or Graeme to come and comfort me, I decided to dig out some more pillows and try to sleep on an angle. It worked somewhat. The dreams shifted to more palatable ones, though still with a slightly nightmarish quality, and a greater volume of sleep time compared with conscious time.

By 5:30 a.m. I was pretty well awake and began to think again of calling doctors, friends, (who do I know that is a nurse?), or family. By 7:00 a.m. I settled on Graeme. So I called and asked for Elizabeth and him to come and visit me. They arrived within a half hour and spent the morning caring for me by reading, praying silently and bringing food and medicine. The medicine was Gravol from my own supply, and I took two to attempt some sleep, but I only dozed a bit before getting out of bed to face the real world.

It is amazing to me now, as I sit here by myself typing, how gradually I shifted from such staggering depression at 7:00 a.m. to my current state of tranquillity by the keyboard. The process was not without its dips.

This was not just another day at the office. I went to the doctor to get the news. Nothing showed up on the MRI leaving Motor Neurone Disease (ALS/Lou Gehrig's) as the most logical possibility. My friend Bill Cozens and I went and picked up his wife Margie at her work and then Bill brought me home. Fraser and I went over there for dinner. We had a great stew and soda biscuits.

Starting a New Life

On April 24, 1996 I wrote in my journal:

> *Today starts a life of new focus. What we already know about ourselves as a renewable, surging, vital resource carried about in a deteriorating vehicle is simply defined in a new way. Just as the time span of physical deterioration*

takes on a somewhat more defined role so should my call to glorify God in my spirit. "Therefore I will boast all the more gladly about my weaknesses, so that Christ's power may rest on me. That is why, for Christ's sake, I delight in weaknesses, in insults, in hardships, in persecutions, in difficulties. For when I am weak, then I am strong" (2Cor 12:9–10). This morning I am reading Luke 5 and it is full of healing. I will call for healing only that God might be glorified... not that I might escape hardship.

Whether healed or not I will never be the same again. In giving up my accounting practice I feel like I am giving up that part of my life, and now my emphasis will be on Whitewater and finding supplemental income through accounting, bookkeeping and tax returns. And finding time to write and study.

As I reflect now on my journal entries and how I dealt with this cataclysmic bend in the road of life, I am struck with the realization that my emotional state improved as I gradually became adjusted to the reality of my physical condition. I recall saying to myself, when the physical facts became obvious, that if I am to know what my true reaction to this reality is, I need to drop the artificial stimulants. So I did and, although my journal reflects several weeks of traumatic adjustment, I quit the pills and allowed my own spiritual underpinnings to line my path. Reflecting on five years of living with ALS I realize that the worst emotional trauma was during the year that I was unaware of its presence. There is no way of knowing how an earlier diagnosis might have affected my life during that time. But the emotional struggle of dealing with the year's varying issues I have described, the despair that caused my doctor to diagnose me as being in a state of depression and the subsequent period of discovering my illness were by far greater traumas than anything I have experienced since. Proverbs 18:14 says "A man's spirit sustains him in sickness, but a crushed spirit who can bear?" How faith-building it is that the Scripture so consistently reaches in and pinpoints reality.

This is my experience precisely; it is this spirit within me, given to me at birth and injected with power through Jesus, that sustains me. It is when that spirit is stilted, attacked or crushed that we are in desperate straits. Our bodies are doomed anyway, so when they are afflicted it is the natural course. The spirit lives forever, so its condition is vital.

Never the Same Again

"Down" is the word for me today. Getting married; changing jobs; getting immersed in the family business and selling the house—how will I do it all? After talking to Bill Cozens about the options for the house, I decided to call Lynne for another go-round. Final, final, final confirmation that under no circumstances would she want to live in this house. I think I really wanted to hear that again. Each time I do I am able to commit more to the alternatives...maybe.

In Sickness and in Health

Last Sunday, "church" was tough—I was on the verge of tears throughout. How much of this is just feeling sorry for myself. Rick Van R. and I went for lunch and left church while communion was still winding up. As I left, David Ducklow came up to me to give me a hug and I broke into tears in his arms. I didn't try to explain anything. I just carried on with Rick. We went to the Cactus Club where Karen was waiting on tables, and Karen and I had a good chat about the house.

I stained more of the bathroom last night, getting it ready for sale. Kyle called to arrange a meeting with me to discuss "the house." I will do it. Tuesday night. Fraser's birthday is next, so I need to arrange a gift. Probably I will just give him a final $500. From July 1, he will be somewhat on his own. I keep having discussions with him about how he is about to take on responsibility for more of his life's decisions. It is hard to see this final break-up of our family looming like a blind curve. What is around the bend?

> *This morning I woke with a definite feeling of weakness in my legs and fear in the pit of my stomach. As usual getting out of bed is the answer. The desire to have Lynne beside me in these times is enormous. Five weeks tonight we will be at the Briars—our wedding place in Ontario—God willing. I sure do hope I don't go downhill a lot before then.*

I decided to grab one of my many "daily devotionals." I have dozens it seems but could only find one. That's enough. It was Richard Swindoll's, *The Finishing Touch*. I read about how he watched his last child, with bride attached, accelerate out of the church parking lot on a Harley, and then how he reflects on 37 years of his own marriage. He refers to a book, *Passages of Marriage*, where a "fifth and final stage" of marriage is described as "Transcendent Love—a profound and peaceful perspective toward your partner and toward life." I guess it's easy for authors to write stuff like that on the assumption that everything goes according to plan. I may or may not reach 37 years of marriage but if I do it will be with two different brides—one gone after 29 years of marriage and then life with Lynne, the one I get to spend the "Transcendent Love" time with. But it is filled with uncertainty.

It is September now. I have just finished mowing the back lawn because the rains are coming and no one who lives at 180 Carisbrooke seems to notice that some of it is four inches high. It was a tough go (I had to clean the mower out about ten times) but, though I'm asking myself why I'm doing it, it is an opportunity to mow a lawn one more time. Maybe it will be my last. There is no reason why Fraser or Karen would see mowing the lawn as an exciting opportunity that might never happen again. The house will be sold and I am losing strength.

But selling the house will not be that simple. Lynne has declared unequivocally that she will not live in the house. But developments after the wedding would make selling the house more complicated than I could have dared imagine.

Initially, we had set our wedding date at September 28. This would have resulted in getting married within days of the first anniversary of our meeting. But the introduction of this new dynamic initiated the advancement of the date. And so it was that on July 6, 1996 in St. George's Anglican Church, Campbellville, Ontario, I for the second time and Lynne for the first, vowed that we would commit our lives to one another, in sickness and in health, "until death us do part." This time, that particular vow hung in the air like a curtain, daring us to look beyond.

The House that Wouldn't

For Lynne, marrying me was not only taking on a health risk but a business risk. Developments in the family business, Whitewater, were soon to occupy me fully and throttle our intended sale of the house to purchase something that was "ours."

The financial health of an enterprise is measured by various ratios. One important measurement is the current asset ratio, which tells how many current asset dollars there are for each current liability dollar. Obviously a 1:1 ratio would mean that by turning all current assets, such as accounts receivable and inventory into cash, you would be able to pay all current liabilities. At April 30, 1997 our current asset ratio was less than 1:1. In terms of cash capital we were hardly in the position to build a doghouse. Lynne and I had arranged for a two-week holiday in England and Austria in June. I received a $40,000 payment on the sale of my accounting practice, and the cash flow demands of the company drew that small change into its vortex, like sofa lint into a vacuum cleaner. Lynne was not too pleased when I told her what I had done, but I was still optimistic that somehow we would prevail. So we headed for Europe leaving our financial future in the hands of our two oldest children.

I did not expect our fortunes to rise or fall during this two-week period, so I returned with nothing more than the realization that the paper would be piled high and that my deteriorating typing skills would be put to the test entering the mass of data. Two projects were now well underway and the payroll was beginning to climb. Kyle was beginning to perfect the art of claiming the maximum progress draw in the early stages of a project, in order to supplement the cash flow. Although this potentially inflates revenues it establishes cash revenues for the following month. I would enter our progress draw into the system at the end of each month. Initially, of course, with all revenues reported and only invoices from suppliers received to that point entered in the system, the profit looked magnificent. As each day passed in the following month, suppliers' statements would arrive and as invoices were posted the profit line would gradually decline. It was a hand-to-mouth routine as I waited for the final result.

A serious cash crunch was in the immediate forecast.

It was about mid-September when my stomach muscles started to tell me that the blush had come off the rose. Far too much was going on and we were out of control. A commercial neighbour on Craig's job was being extremely objectionable and created inefficiencies by insisting that we not defile the air space above his building with our crane. Further, under no circumstances could we trespass on his property. Both demands were difficult to abide by since the parcels of land shared a common property line. The pressures related to scheduling, cash flow, and personality conflicts on the high-rise project, known as Lord Stanley, were mounting. The symptoms of my disease were progressing, causing me considerable anxiety over my ability to handle the pressure.

There was a strange paradox here. On the one hand, I was convinced that we had the perfect formula for a successful business with the combination of abilities and backgrounds already described. This confidence was reinforced by the two years of growth and success already achieved. On the other hand, we were currently out of control and I had allowed it to happen, risking my capital and putting immeasurable emotional pressure on a physically challenged body. There was no question about who would be required to extricate the business from this mess, if extrication were possible. During the summer, recognizing my own physical limitations and realizing that in the long run my partners would need a financially oriented partner, I began to talk and meet with several business friends with the idea of forming a board of advisers should I become unable to continue in active management. While these discussions were going on, I had increased our line of credit to $150,000, using my residence as security, while our biweekly payrolls began to push $90,000. By late September it was routine for me to call the bank to assure them that although the payroll would cause our overdraft limit to be breached we would have our month-end draw within a couple of days and all would be well. But I knew that all would not be well if there was not a major insertion of capital into this groaning enterprise.

Somehow we managed to hold off our creditors sufficiently to make the October 17 payroll. We were expecting that the bank would cover our October 31 payroll with the knowledge that we would be receiving our next draw on November 3 or 4. They had been fairly compliant to this point. No such luck. On October 29 the bank called our office and informed us that they had withdrawn their automatic debit instructions with the payroll company and that we would need certified checks to cover the October 31 payroll. Failure to meet the payroll would mean our bonding company would have to step in and that would mean disaster.

Through the cloud of stress I rallied myself to admit that I needed some help from some friends. I started phoning. It is difficult to describe the humbling experience it is to ask close friends for this kind of assistance and have some of them take the risk. Within 24 hours I was sitting in the bank boardroom with two friends and their cheque books. One lent us $50,000 and the other $25,000. I managed to drag out another $10,000 from a half forgotten line of credit and $15,000 from my account with my former accounting practice. The immediate crisis was averted. In the following month I was able, thanks to the generosity of my sisters, to replace the money borrowed from my friends with a $100,000 collateral mortgage on their home.

As each miserable day crept by during this October crisis I recall trying to imagine the total sum of anxiety I was yet to experience before this mess was over. I pictured the months of November, December and January as a time vacuum that I was about to be sucked into, until all these uncontrollable factors could be sucked in there with me. But each day was so full of anxiety and each night such an interminable nightmare it was hard to imagine ever being spat out into a normal day again. Some nights I would lie back on the pillow with Lynne and just express the despair I felt. All she could do was hold me.

Here she was, the total newcomer to this family in its headlong pursuit of chaos, and she was totally isolated from any control over what might happen. So she just carried on cooking meals, doing the housework and beginning the long and arduous task of caring for my physical and emotional needs. Her quiet concession to whatever fate was to befall us was a source of strength and optimism. When my appetite disappeared and I suggested that now might be the time to install a feeding tube, she laughed it off with confident good humour, stalling that inevitable move for another two and a half years.

Fortunately, my partners' faith in themselves was well founded and even as the Lord Stanley ground to its agonizing end, we were starting a project which would result in sufficient profit by our April 30 fiscal year-end to reduce our operating loss to $30,000. Within a year our borrowed capital was repaid. The house was sold and a condominium unit bought. In two years we moved from virtual insolvency to modest but self-sustaining liquidity. My sons' vision and giftedness had turned this learning experience into a fruitful business. I was delighted with Whitewater.

Springtime and Fall Laced Together

Although we are free to attempt to divine God's purpose, we will never succeed in doing so. The reason is that we cannot know (the manifest contradictions are too disturbing) what is behind particular phenomena and therefore must make do with only the grandest plan of God, which deals with eternal salvation. Our burden is to keep the faith: to do this (the grammar of assent) requires the discipline of submission, some assurance that those who are stricken can, even so, be happy; and that the greatest tonic of all is divine love, which is nourished by human love, even as human love is nourished by divine love.

William F. Buckley, *Nearer, My God*

If happiness can be calibrated separately from differing facets of our lives, I can say I'm happier in most ways than I have ever been.

I venture out on the deck on a Saturday morning that was designed for the start of all spring clean-ups. Blue skies that blow the budding trees into eye sockets shimmering with reflections of pruning shears. Green mould rimming into the sunny patches from the shady strips along walls and fences, inviting the bark and misty bite of the pressure washing machine. Meanwhile the hum of various motorized tools float in the tangy air as an announcement of the start of the handyman's and gardener's joint declaration of war on weed and wood.

I stood there like a kid in a video arcade with folding money in my pocket but nowhere to make change. The atmosphere was trenchant with an intoxicating brew but I could only smell and not drink. The industrious sounds of house-building at the corner. The wisteria bush clamouring for a serious trim. The deck underfoot needing a scrub and a wash and the flower boxes pleading for rejuvenation. Lonely sticks of lumber lying beside the railing that were intended as extensions of the trellis.

Thanksgiving and Remembrance

What an amazing year. While I grappled with declining health the Lord had been wondrously gentle with me. Let me count the ways to praise:

1. Lynne, Lynne, Lynne.
2. Whitewater recovery. Exactly a year since I started to lose serious sleep.
3. Tom Gamet came with his son and did a bunch of repair work.
4. Randy came and painted the house.
5. Tim came and provided new life and this year even a bit of room money.
6. Cash flow has worked.
7. Eugene Peterson's teaching.
8. Great reading.

9. Fraser's progress in flying.
10. Karen's progress in school and life.
11. I can still walk.
12. I can still talk.
13. The encouragement of ALS people.

It is November 11, 1998—Remembrance Day—full of images of old men still marching to defiant tunes with heads high and hearts humbled in the memory of the broken bodies that fell around them over 80 years ago. My impression is that if you survived it you survived it whole, at least physically, unlike Vietnam, where you could lose pieces and still have to come home to make the best of what was left.

Henri Nouwen says our life is a series of losses. We are born and lose the security of the womb (though that doesn't seem too secure these days). We graduate from high school and lose most of our friends. We find a job and lose our freedom. We die and lose it all.

Those of us who wake each day with fresh reminders of the limitations of our bodies look for affirmation that, though our body is assaulted, our spirit is not crushed. The deterioration of bodily function brings greater and greater dependence on others, but the loss of independent physical activity gives us the time to ponder the relationship between body and soul.

Henri Nouwen's years of experience working with severely handicapped and terminally ill patients and the simultaneous occurrence of the death of his friends and thoughts of his aging father, caused him to write *Our Greatest Gift*, a short meditation on "dying and caring" as he sought to "befriend death." Clearly his perspective is based on the eternalistic view of Christianity in the life and teachings of Christ. But his perspective is infused with experience, not dogmatism, and any reader, regardless of their faith or lack of it, will warm to his expressions of hope and love.

Nouwen applies the principle that we are all children of God and within that common ground we begin and end our lives totally dependent on others. "The mystery of life is that we discover this human togetherness not when we are powerful and strong, but when we are vulnerable and weak." Then, using his own experiences, Nouwen builds a case for choosing to use our final days to build a legacy of a generous and thankful spirit with those who care for us.

For those who provide care for the terminally ill, Nouwen suggests there is an issue of choosing. Choosing between fighting against the inevitable or accepting that our increasing dependence on others is a gateway to God's grace. Mortality is common to all of us. When caregivers give up the desire to cure, their care "can truly heal in ways far beyond our dreams and expectations."

We all look for ways to turn the tide of our body's misfortune to our soul's advantage. Due to our ties to this world and the mist that obscures the next one, we find that a very difficult task. Nouwen's book focuses on the destination and sheds light on the path so that the cared-for and the caregiver are both illuminated on the way.

Bold with our experience of Remembrance Day we were lured south by a chunk of blue over Georgia Strait that looks more like the sunroof of a very large car than a serious change in the weather. The radio reported someone lost in the rain swollen Capilano river in a kayaking accident and we could see the activity of Search and Rescue at the mouth of the river, as we headed for Third Beach for a walk on the seawall and a circuit of Lost Lagoon. I didn't know this guy (who turns out to be a 50-year-old well-known Vancouver nature photographer) but this tragedy stood up against my own in some strange way. I'm losing my life gradually; he lost his in an instant. I lost my ability to kayak during the last year or so; his ability to kayak killed him. This was too nice a day for either of us to be dying, but somehow I will be very content in my perambulations over the puddles and wet leaves and by the silky waters of English Bay where so much living is taking place, yet so near to where this life was lost.

Graduating To A Chair

We brought the push chair to Regent College where Lynne and I are registered for a conference, "Treasures in the Attic: Theological Resources for Evangelical Spirituality Today." I gauged the distance from the handicap parking space to the lecture hall and decided to walk. After the morning's double dose of academic theorizing on "The Quest for Community & Spirituality," and "Renewing the Heart and Mind: Sapiential Theology and Spiritual Formation" we ran into a living fleshed-out example of what these lofty themes could only conjecture: Jenny Armerding with her two sons Malcolm and Dana, both seriously handicapped. Jenny has cared for both for several years and recently secured legal adoption as a single mother. By the standards of our society this doesn't look wise at all, but by Christ's reasoning, which turned most of our wisdom to mush, her actions are the heart of "true spirituality." "When you did it for the least of these you did it for me" (Matt 25:40).

Dana knew that I was about to graduate to a power chair and was interested in my progress in that direction. He initiated conversation at lunch and we experienced "community and spirituality."

> *I have now graduated to a scooter. I am on a roll—first trip to Costco on the scooter. This system beats walking any day. All I lack is a bigger basket on the front and the motivation to buy. I desire neither.*
>
> *A faint glow of solar radiation mocked our repose. Golf, glowing green on the video screen, was changing heroes and my favorite was down and almost out. "Queen Elizabeth Park," I said, between swings, "the blossoms may be out." We had taken a walk at Kits point earlier in the week where the flowering trees had jump-started our springtime optimism. But the shrubs and plants of Little Mountain had either not been paying attention to the calendar or were simply intimidated by the persistently low snow line on the North Shore mountains. Only the daffodils dared to show a ruddy cheek to the final throes of winter. It was cold enough to send us inside the observatory and a walk through the Plexiglas dome protected from the early spring of 49 degrees of latitude.*
>
> *The summer now has come and gone. The family home of almost three decades has gone. More muscle and personal energy has gone.*

In between getting up and going to bed I kept asking myself the question, "How did I get into this mess?" I guess the only difference is that before I had ALS I had no shortage of people telling me why I was in a mess, and they would do it for free. Now, people are spending millions of dollars trying to figure out why I'm so screwed up and they still have no idea.

Kissing a Moving Target

This may be hard for some to believe but women find me incredibly attractive. Maybe they have a natural affinity for people who look helpless. At church, women are always coming up to me to give me a kiss. Maybe they feel safe because they know I can't grope. For some reason they always come at me from the left side where the controls for my power chair are located. Inevitably, just as their lips touch down, so does their coat, or purse, or hips touch down on my toggle-switch which starts sending me and my chair backwards. They have no idea what's happening so they keep trying to reach me as I become a moving target. Meanwhile I'm yelling,"Hold it!" as I try to shut off the power. It's kind of like trying to bite into one of those large candy apples: you get your mouth over it and your teeth projected and the whole thing slips away from you.

As ALS steals your strength and flexibility you depend more and more on others to take care of your basic needs. There is nothing more basic than the regular need to urinate and defecate. The circle of friends and family that have been, on occasion, recruited to assist in these matters grows gradually larger and my two oldest boys were in the loop early. On one occasion, after our third trip to the urinal in a local pub where Craig had assisted me in extracting and redepositing my equipment, I broke down in tears right in the bathroom. So there we were: son consoling father right in the middle of a public lavatory.

Not much later my other son Kyle was helping me in a theatre wash room. Normally I would use the handicapped stall but this time I suggested we just belly up to the urinal. I ran my chair up to the nearest porcelain receptacle, lifted my foot supports, and stood to perform. No sooner had I begun than Kyle, trying to be as helpful as possible by holding my arm, started dragging his coat over the control toggle on my power chair, which we had neglected to turn off, rotating the leg supports that caught my ankles as they went and pushed me sideways. I started screaming to Kyle to stop it while he yelled back that he wasn't doing anything. I grabbed the top of the urinal to save myself just as Kyle figured out what he was doing. The trauma of it closed up my passages. We regrouped, and fled the scene, leaving numerous patrons of the facility scratching their heads (assuming that they had hands free to do so).

Recently Kyle was assisting me in our bathroom at home and as I stood watching the action in the mirror, along with the reflection of this very large son, I marveled that his spiritual and bodily origins made their entry into the world by means of this same bodily member. Fortunately for him, I wasn't in the bathroom when "it" happened. (Note: what deviant channel in my intellect causes me to make these kinds of observations?)

But now I have arrived at the stage where I need help for the whole procedure. So I have an expanding cast of family and friends who have had to get closer to me than they ever had a right to expect. But it's very interesting to observe the difference between men and women when it comes to facing the music. When one of my male friends was gingerly helping me extract my weapon I observed to him that women just go right at it. They reach in and pull it out like it was a sausage they were about to skin. The men reach in like they were about to steal a piece of meat from an alligator.

Thinking About My Death

I have been reading *Measuring The Days* by Walter Wangerin. His scripture reference for the day is Ecc 7:1–7:

> "*A good name is better than fine perfume,*
> *and the day of death better than the day of birth.*
> *It is better to go to a house of mourning*
> *than to go to a house of feasting,*
> *for death is the destiny of everyone;*
> *the living should take this to heart.*"

How does this square with the tape given to me by a friend? The tape offers rejuvenated health through "nutriceuticals"? It sounds as though they offer eternal life in a bottle and you become a millionaire at the same time through multi-level marketing as you offer it to others. "It will sell itself!" they imply, and why wouldn't it with those results?

So I have set out to memorize Revelation chapter 5—the soothing cadence of the inspired Word. Would I be filling my brain cells with them if they were working "properly"? No. But visions of the Lamb of God at the centre of the throne and the four beasts and the twenty-four elders bowing down fill my head instead of the specter of an irate client tearing a strip off me for not planning his tax payments properly. As a child I remember the story of August van Ryn memorizing scripture because he was going blind. Can I be resolved enough to stockpile these treasures to be mined over and over again when I don't have the energy to turn the pages of a book?

I finished reading *The Heart of the Matter* by Graham Greene. Scobie, the protagonist, has gone to borrow a medical book from his bank manager in order to research the symptom of angina. He is planning his suicide. Robinson is unusually cheerful compared to his normal anxiety over health issues, and suggests that Scobie go see Dr. Travis at the Argyle Hospital. As far as his own problem is concerned he says, "I'm not bothered about it anymore. The truth of the matter is, Scobie, I'm…." But Scobie is so intent on reading the medical book that Robinson never finishes the sentence and is then interrupted by Scobie saying that perhaps he'll see Travis. "I hope he cheers me up as he's done you."

"Well, my case," the manager said evasively, "had peculiar features."

Scobie then goes to visit his boss, the Commissioner, where he discovers that Robinson has two years to live, and muses, "I suppose that is what comes of knowing the worst—one is left alone with the worst and it is like peace" and recalls his conversation: "I hope we all die as calmly." Full of guilt, Scobie will take his own life a few days later.

I don't know what the source of Robinson's peace was but I identify with him. When I heard my medical diagnosis a lot of struggles ceased. Planning was easier. There were fewer questions to answer and fewer uncertainties that mattered. Maybe if Scobie knew he had only two years to live he would have purged his guilt and enjoyed life for the time he had.

It is only a coincidence that I strap on my microphone (on my voice-activated computer), two years after reading this, to reflect some more on my death. Robinson would now be dead but I still plug along. I am two years closer, as everyone is, and I contemplate more the narrowing scope of my life as debility takes a firmer grip on my perspective.

> *So I increasingly turn to the soothing phrases of Scripture. It is a miracle how words that so perfectly describe my flagging physical fortunes can raise my spirits rather than lower them. I suppose it is the ability to identify with someone else's sorrow. In this case it is both the Psalmist and the Lord himself.*
>
> *"I am poured out like water, and all my bones are out of joint. My heart has turned to wax; it has melted away within me. My strength is dried up like a potsherd, and my tongue sticks to the roof of my mouth; you lay me in the dust of death. Dogs have surrounded me; a band of evil men has encircled me, they have pierced my hands and my feet. I can count all my bones; people stare and gloat over me. They divide my garments among them and cast lots for my clothing. But you, O LORD, be not far off; O my Strength, come quickly to help me" (Psalm 22:14–19).*

What a great mystery it is that, 400 years before Christ, his suffering could be so accurately described so that, despite its mocking accuracy of my own condition, it brings strength because of its identity with him. I suffer the conditions of one verse—"My strength is dried up like a potsherd, and my tongue sticks to the roof of my mouth." Jesus suffered them all. Then the cry, "you, O Lord… my strength!" becomes a reality just by taking in the text. Which I did.

Laughing and Crying My Way To Heaven

Hope is the Thing With Feathers
That perches in the soul
And sings the tune without the words
And Never Stops
At All...

Emily Dickinson

I recall my father naming the random bad things that happen to us as "the vicissitudes of life." In the world of limited vocabulary people just say, "Shit happens." But when it does we are able to overcome because of love.

Getting a "G" Tube

The world moves on outside my window under a clear blue sky. Our new home overlooks the Capilano canyon. The evergreens in our valley are reflecting the sun in my window and a slight wind moves their branches in the same way I clearly remember when we first came here last August 1999. They will be reflecting a different light when I return in a few days depending on the time and weather. But I will be somehow different once again. Today I go to the hospital and the medicine men move in to insert the tube that will siphon supplementary energy into this screwed-up body. They are going to punch a hole in my stomach wall and pull a tube, with a washer on the end, out through the opening. To do this from the inside out, they first stick a flashlight on a wire down my throat to find the hole and pull a string up through it to attach to the tube. (One more step on the road to greater dependence). Trees die I know. They get disease like the rest of us. But the ones outside my window look like they will last forever drawing nourishment up through their roots, leaves, and needles in some simple predefined way. I guess I'm lucky. When trees get sick they cut them down. Too often they do it even when they're not.

Done. Barely fifteen minutes under the knife and I can fill my tank like you would a broken down coupe: fuel siphoned in from a plastic bag three times a day. The procedure took less than twenty minutes to complete and since I was only partly sedated I could feel the various appliances being run up and down my throat. Later that evening in my hospital room, as the first can of complementary formula dripped into my previously vacuated stomach cavity, Lynne suggested I proceed with preparation for sacking out by brushing my teeth. The realization that this was possible while I was still "eating" started the production of the **"Top 10 advantages of having a G-tube."** By the time I hit the sack we had composed four or five of them and I added a couple more when I woke up during the night. The list was completed at home after two nights in the hospital. Here they are in their final form:

10. You can brush your teeth while you eat.
9. You can drink all you want and still be able to say "alcohol never touches my lips."
8. You can eat brussels sprouts and never need to smell them.
7. You can eat at McDonald's and never have to taste the food.
6. You have twice the belly button lint.
5. You can talk with your bag full.
4. You can eat at Hooters and the waitresses stare at YOU!
3. You never have to complain that the food isn't hot enough.
2. It gives the term "body piercing" a whole new meaning.
1. When you wash out the system you get to drink your own dish water.

We subscribe to an electronic digest on the Internet devoted to ALS issues. People write their stories, ask questions, appeal for help, sell medical appliances and offer opinions. After posting the "Top 10" on the Digest I received at least twenty responses thanking me for offering the lighter side of this further invasion of our privacy. Several people involved in various aspects of health care, asked permission to use the list in newsletters or to post in their offices. I, of course, said yes, having already dedicated this bit of nonsense to the public domain.

The Pain of Endings

Last night Craig took me to the movie, "Cider House Rules." As it wound up I began to cry and wondered why. The ending, with Homer Wells going back to the orphanage, had an element of emotion. But I concluded that the real reason for my modest breakdown was that one more thing was ending. The event, being with Craig, was ending and every ending now seems to result in a climax of emotion. As shortness of breath signals shortness of life, I see each encounter with each child, once it is over, as a depletion of opportunity to enjoy, in person, the love I feel for each of them. Earlier in the week all of us, except Karen and R.J., were at the St. James Wells pub in Coquitlam and after I was in the van, Fraser came by the window to say goodnight and tell me he would be over to see us before he leaves for his flying job up north. I was already on the edge of a chin pucker, the first stage of a total face dissolve, thinking about another social ending when he started reminding me of a much more significant termination, his 21-year homestand. He saw my facial contortions. I told him to "get out of here," and I think he understood. It is an ending that will be hard to bear. He leaves Saturday and plans to be up there for six months. It is great for him but not something I like thinking about. I feel the compression of time and that old paradox, the sweet sense of sorrow.

> *Another Easter weekend has come and I have one more opportunity to divert the image of my suffering self to the one who suffered for us all. Yesterday, in our Good Friday service, we were reminded of the seven instances where Christ spoke from the cross. The first one was, "Forgive them for they know not what they do." It was a final confirmation of what he taught us when he told us how to pray: "Forgive us our sins, for we also forgive everyone who sins against us" (Luke 11:4).*

It reminds me of what I must also say from my weak and helpless position as I look at the atrocities committed by society at every level: "Forgive them for they know not what they do." What other hope do we have than to live in forgiveness? What other hope do we have in death than to believe the testimony of those who saw, on that Easter morning, Jesus alive but with the marks of the cross on his body?

We have, in our church, a tradition for Easter services. On Good Friday we write on a small piece of paper the thought, desire, trespass, prayer or emotion that we wish to leave at Christ's cross. Each person walks to a cross, which has been erected at the front, and places their inscription in one of the small holes that have been drilled in it. On Easter Sunday each piece of paper is replaced with a daffodil. While my hardened instincts squirm a bit at this hint of sentimentality I told Lynne to write on my piece of paper "my weakness" and when I tried to say it I broke down. How many times have I called out to God to heal me yet I am like the Apostle Paul who recounts in his second letter to the Corinthians, chapter 12:

> *"Three times I pleaded with the Lord to take it away from me. But he said to me, 'My grace is sufficient for you, for my power is made perfect in weakness.' Therefore I will boast all the more gladly about my weaknesses, so that Christ's power may rest on me. That is why, for Christ's sake, I delight in weaknesses, in insults, in hardships, in persecutions, in difficulties. For when I am weak, then I am strong" (vv. 8–10).*

This is the reality that Jesus lived so perfectly. The power to overcome death was only accomplished because he was weak on the cross. We all fight our weaknesses; we don't want them. Weakness counteracts the power and control we desire for our lives, reducing our options. This is not to say that it is bad to be strong, just that we have very little control about how much strength we have. When confronted with weakness, strengths are created and events are shaped in ways which are never possible by sheer power. Simply look at what Jesus accomplished by being led meekly to the cross and, by contrast, consider what happened to the Roman Empire which carried out the execution.

This is easier to write about than it is to live.

My Sixtieth Birthday Extravaganza

My birthday extravaganza, was carefully planned by Lynne and my friends. As mentioned before I did my Superman entrance. The evening proceeded with much laughter and delight. But when I'd thought about delivering a serious heart-felt speech I knew I'd have trouble, so I wrote the "unspeakable speech" and we handed it out to all who wanted it.

Most of you will know that I feel more comfortable speaking to you "off the cuff" than from a script. But when I stop making jokes and start thinking about either the losses I feel or the blessings I experience, emotion takes over and I am unable to speak. So I will save you the tears and communicate by carefully constructed sentences on a plain sheet of paper. I can safely say, even though I write this in advance, that this has been the absolutely best day of my sixty-first year.

So here are some sentiments that are a little too deep for me to speak.

1. One of the outcomes of sickness and weakness is that you discover and experience the care of the people around you. My care givers include doctors, nurses,

Vancouver hospital ALS clinic people, British Columbia ALS society staff, North Shore health care workers, friends, family and, finally, my wife. I see every act of kindness as God's promise contained in Jesus' words, ***"blessed are the poor in spirit for they shall see God."*** *When we are strong and independent we can miss this lavish expression of God's love.*

2. My life has been filled with the blessing of children. Psalm 127 says,

> ***Sons [and daughters] are a heritage from the LORD, children a reward from him.***
>
> ***Like arrows in the hands of a warrior are sons [and daughters] born in one's youth. Blessed is the man whose quiver is full of them. They will not be put to shame when they contend with their enemies in the gate (vv. 3–5).***

As our children are now facing this same enemy at the gate for the second time they demonstrate the reality of this encouragement from the Psalms to face the tough things in life and keep moving. They are the ultimate reward and encouragement for Lynne and me.

> ***3. "The glory of Friendship is not the outstretched hand, nor the kindly smile, nor the joy of companionship; it is the spiritual inspiration that comes to one when he discovers that someone else believes in him and is willing to trust him with their friendship. My friends have come unsought. The great God gave them to me" (Ralph Waldo Emerson).***

You have come to me, unsought, through the events that occasion a life of 60 years. You have greeted me, encouraged me, taught me, prayed for me, corrected me and cheered me. You have laughed at my jokes, accepted my antics, and overlooked my peculiarities. You have loved my wives and encouraged and taught my children. And much more than that is hidden but not lost in the mist of time. These memories are a symphony to my senses and I can't get the headphones off.

4. Finally I want to acknowledge the fabulous gift that God has given me, my wife, Lynne. Our meeting and falling in love was a miracle to me, but the greater miracle is that she sees it as one as well. Her care for me is beyond measure. Not only is it consistent every day but it is filled with her personal joy. You have experienced that joy tonight but I receive it every day. Thank you, Lynne, for your love and for this great party.

I finished up my monologue by describing the implications of my G-tube and having our master of ceremonies and friend, Gord Taylor, read my "Top 10" advantages of having a G-tube.

The party wound down with music and dancing. I had asked Kyle to include Anne Murray's, "Can I Have This Dance for the Rest of our Lives," and when it came on, my daughter, Karen, and I found each other's eyes. She climbed onto my knee and I swirled my chair around the floor to carry on a short tradition, started only months before, that this song would be ours for the rest of our lives.

As the building chilled appreciably with all the doors open for the exit of guests and the removal of equipment, my feet and shin bones sucked up the frigid air like smoke to salmon. One of our friends had given me a small quilt as a birthday gift and this was wrapped around my pillaged pins as I headed out the door for home. It took a week to recover.

Off to Camp

The next adventure for my frail faculties was a six-day visit in the palliative care ward of Lions Gate Hospital. The occasion was a bit of respite for Lynne while she went to Toronto for our niece's wedding. We had attempted to obtain space in a long term care facility through our local home care contact but found that there was no space available until July. The second option, lining up 24-hour home care, just seemed to be an enormous chore, so I called the head of palliative care. I knew that they had essentially closed their doors to ALS people because they had been saddled with someone on a respirator for two years and feared that all of us sorry souls with this weird disease would cause them the same distress. My years of involvement with the Hospice Society made me familiar with the issue and since we had already decided that I would not follow the respirator route, I felt confident in pleading my case. They gave me my "green card" which gives me access to palliative care whenever I need it so, as Lynne put it, "I was off to camp."

"Camp" would possibly be a harsh description of my experience but one element of that analogy does fit. Every camp has its misfit and I was it. Palliative care patients are almost exclusively cancer sufferers, and most are physically able to move about or are totally confined to bed. Much of the care is centred in pain control and comfort in bed. By contrast, my needs are almost totally in the area of physical assistance—getting into bed, out of bed, eating, peeing, pooping, dressing, undressing. Beyond these normal daily activities was the need to connect my BiPap machine at night and connect my G-tube every mealtime. Of course the nurses changed shift every twelve hours, so each one needed to be taught each function and to be made aware of the degree of my physical needs.

It was exhausting. The simple procedure that Lynne and I follow at home when moving from power chair to toilet and back with all the necessary accomplishments in between, became a new adventure with each new nurse almost every time. Once, I had three nurses lifting me off the can to set me on my feet with my hands stationed on the arms of my chair, at which point it is customary for my lucky assistant to clear away the residue of the just completed function. But there was no appropriate material available to do so which meant that I was required to stand there while one of the nurses left to fetch some. By the time I was sitting in my chair again I was sucking major air. It took a good three minutes of steady heavy breathing to recover sufficiently to reach the controls and get myself out of the john.

The Search for the Perfect Catheter

The most significant area of physical and mental fatigue, however, resulted from attempts to establish a viable living relationship between me and a condom catheter. We had been considering for some time that the use of this unique device would simplify my life when I am away from home for the afternoon or evening. Anyway, with my being in palliative care pampered by an unlimited supply of nurses, we thought it would be a great chance to try a condom catheter. The idea of whizzing on demand sounded like a dream so I recruited some nurses to hook me up—a continuous plastic hose securely attached to my penis and running downhill to a bag on my ankle. What could possibly go wrong?

The first urge came upon me while I was in conversation with some friends in the lounge. Aha! I said to myself, this is kind of scary but they'll never know I'm peeing right in the middle of their sentence. There is already some trauma involved as you let go in the middle of someone's story, but the sense of hopelessness and fear that hits you when you realize you are warm in places you ought not to be is difficult to describe. Your hands want to cover the damage and your eyes want to see the evidence but you don't move any of them. You're frozen eye to eye with your storyteller but your concentration is following your urine and you're still not sure if it's going into the bag or into your pants. This feeling must be normal, you say to yourself. Professional nurses installed this thing. Then you peek. You have already shut it off but the damage is done so you lean forward with your forearms over your knees and politely nod in agreement while your mind races over escape options.

Why is it that doctors can tap into your heart and run your blood through a machine and put it back in your body but nobody can figure out how to build a foolproof condom? With four separate attempts in the hospital, none worked perfectly.

When I got back home we arranged for a home care nurse to come and demonstrate the perfect installation. I will protect her good name by giving her the alias of Florence. Florence and my wife and I congregated in the bathroom to begin work. After a few attempts by Florence to make some progress, she asked if I have any trouble getting an erection. I said, "not normally but I've never sat exposed in a bathroom with two women before and I'm mighty surprised I don't have one now."

She said, "Well it would help to have a bit of one to get this on."

I said, "One thing I can tell you for sure, I don't have a switch I can use to turn it off half way through." Finally she was able to roll the device on, to some satisfaction, at which point she advised that in order for the glue to adhere she had to grab my member in a full hand-hold, which she proceeded to do. She got a very quick answer to the erection question.

In spite of all Florence's efforts, her condom catheter came off before I even had a chance to use it. We finally found a product that worked but it cost three bucks a pop rather than a dollar—wouldn't you know it. So I don't know if it's because I want to save money or what, but I'll be darned if I'm going to give up on Florence. She's coming back as many times as it takes to get her to perfect her system.

Ready for the Next Dip in the Road

One thing for sure about this disease is that you have to be ready for each new dip in the road. As I mentioned, a big move about a month ago was getting a G-tube installed. I guess one of the things that a doctor writes on the chart for the nurses is that my swallowing is compromised. Of course, all of the nurses assume that means I can't swallow. I was feeling pretty uncomfortable and asked for a couple of Tylenol. The nurse came in with the pills and said, "I guess you need these in a suppository."

I said, "That would be okay with me but isn't that a lot of extra trouble for you?" She looked a little puzzled until I explained to her that I could swallow okay. So I had to train all the nurses so that they wouldn't bring me my pills with their rubber gloves already on.

It occurred to me in the process that the word that is used for a device that is administered in this way is completely misused. "Suppository." Just think of it. This word would be perfect to describe a bank deposit that was supposed to have been made yesterday. The accountant goes to his boss and says "I did a suppository." It even has an apologetic tone. I'm sorry. It was supposed to have gone in yesterday. But the deposit didn't get done until today. "Suppository." It's a perfectly good word and look what it got relegated to.

Debility makes travelling difficult. Considering a trip by air to Toronto, I called Canadian Airlines to find out what it would cost for a business class ticket. The shocking answer came back—$3,600. After catching my breath I asked what I would get for that kind of money over a regular ticket. She described the luxurious seats, the free drinks and the menu selections. I asked her if there is any more insurance that my surviving family members would get if the plane crashed. She kind of snickered and admitted that there wasn't. So I concluded that was just too much money for some personal luxuries.

Now if they had a system for the business class section, where if the plane started to go down, they could close off both ends, have helicopter rotors go out and the whole business section be lifted out and dropped down into the parking lot of the closest Holiday Inn... now that would be worth the extra money.

Thinking About Heaven

When you have a terminal illness you tend to think a bit

about what comes next. Of course, as a Christian, you take some considerable comfort from the promises of Scripture. But you must admit that the total concept of heaven is a little bit vague. There are suggestions of cities with streets paved with gold, angels, a new heaven and new earth, and being with Jesus in Paradise. But what does that look like? So I have been asking the opinion of a few friends:

I asked Arven Eggert—(a guy who has moved at least ten times during his married life) he said heaven will be like a huge residential subdivision with high-rises, townhouses, apartments and single-family homes with big wide streets joining them all together. And everyone will have their own moving van. Every once in a while everyone will move from one location to another.

I asked Doug Norton. Doug likes to sleep in a lot. He just said he was really concerned that somewhere he read in the Bible that there was no night there.

I asked Ralph Bagshaw (career high school counsellor)—he said everyone will be given 24 troubled teenagers to look after.

I asked Marilyn (whose husband, Ralph, has pretty firm opinions on issues that matter to him)—she said that all women would be married to men who have no opinions on anything. When I told her that it was my understanding that there won't be any marriages in heaven she said, "Oh, that would be even better."

I asked Paul Stevens (the author of numerous books on Christian living)—he said that everything in heaven will happen exactly the way everything is explained in his books.

So I'm really none the wiser.

Many of us will spend our lives paying off a mortgage on our home feeling that once this is done we will have attained the comfort-zone which will eliminate much of the need to toil and sweat and allow us a trouble free old age. We may have varying sized pocketbooks or paychecks and our earthly mansions may vary in the number of rooms they contain but we all see them as places of comfort and refuge.

At the other end of the scale what could be worse than to be in trouble and have no place to go? Recently our TV screens have been filled with images of people in deep trouble and no place to go—a traffic jam heading away from the Southern East Coast of the U.S.; people fleeing a hurricane which is about to destroy their homes; Mexicans standing knee deep in water flowing through their streets and washing away entire towns; people in Turkey and Taiwan left homeless by earthquakes; and Kosovars returning to bombed out villages.

Though homeless himself, Jesus recognized how the offering of a real place to dwell would be a comforting image for those in trouble. "In my Father's house are many rooms; if it were not so, I would have told you. I am going there to prepare a place for you" (John 14:2). He used the analogy of a home with many rooms to comfort his disciples as they saw their earthly security dissolving.

As someone who suffers from a terminal illness, I have spent some time considering eternal options. I find myself constructing images of places and activities on this earth and transposing them into some mystical heavenly context—playing golf or soccer. Then I think—darn—we won't be competitive. I dream of building things with my hands—then I think again—what will we need to build things for? Jesus has already prepared everything. But as long as our awareness is limited by our senses it is impossible to imagine how our soul could live outside of our current environment.

Here, I'm going to use a direct quote from an author whose name I forget. This description of eternal mystery has been very helpful to me.

> *Jesus tells how he will go before the disciples into a spiritual realm unseen by them in order to prepare a place for them in a realm of reality that the ego in its fledgling state, limited as it is to sense impression and ego awareness, cannot perceive. This spiritual realm of which Jesus speaks is, in fact, only apprehensible through inner experience such as visions and ecstatic experiences, like the experience Paul describes in 2Corinthians 12: 1–4, in which he tells of being caught up into Paradise and hearing things that cannot be put into any ordinary human language. As long as our consciousness is limited to the information brought us by our physical senses and by our limited ego consciousness, we tend to live in anxiety for we feel alone and unaided and therefore not able to cope with life's threats and problems. Jesus' prescription for this anxiety is faith in him, which also means faith in the reality of another world ordinarily unseen by us.*

This same author goes on to point out that the word "hope" is not used here. Hope relates to how things will turn out for us in this world and we are often disappointed by the outcome. I am involved in a business with my two oldest sons. Our principal work is building concrete structures. Currently we are involved in building a convention centre at the Bayshore Inn. I have faith that every working day both Kyle and Craig are down at the site constructing that building. That faith is based on my experience over the past five years. They bid on the work; they hire employees and they build the building. I hope that we will make a profit doing it. I hope that no one will be injured during construction. But my faith that Kyle and Craig will do it is based on my experience. My faith is in things that are certain. My hope is in the uncertain areas. The dictionary defines faith as "confident belief" and I have confident belief that Jesus is preparing a place for me. My confidence is based on my belief that everything he said he would do, he did. And everything that he said he was, he is.

So in John 14 Jesus emphasizes the point that he and his father are one and Jesus continuously connects himself with the Father's wishes. He wants us to accept with *faith* that reality. But then he gives us a *second option:* if we can't by faith believe in Jesus as one with the Father, then at least believe in the evidence of the miracles that he has done: "Believe me when I say that I am in the Father and the Father is in me; or at least believe on the evidence of the miracles themselves" (John 14:11). But it is pretty clear that he sees this second option as a less than perfect one.

If I were suddenly healed, some of my friends, even my church friends, would possibly doubt that I was really very sick to start with. Others might argue that the medication that I take finally kicked in. But let's assume that the miracle is verified and everyone is justifiably amazed. We would all personally have some verifiable evidence that God answers our prayers for healing. Someone might be convinced through the healing that Jesus is God incarnate and begin to follow him. There certainly would be some major turmoil going on in the local ALS medical community and there would no doubt be a flurry of people with infirmities seeking the source of what had happened so that they too might be healed.

But what would be the effect on our personal daily walk with the Lord? I suggest, very little. I suggest that my healing would have less effect upon others than the arrival of a dear friend at our doorstep to help us deal with a problem that we thought was beyond our ability to handle. Less than the effect of having your spouse tell you they love you. Less than the effect of having Mike Nichols and Jake Penner come and build a bookcase for them, which they did recently for me.

Acts of love—that's what these are and they are the "greater things" Jesus said his disciples would do (John 14:12) and they come through the community of praying, Spirit-filled believers. They are people who walk together following Jesus on the path to the Father and in obedience to the call to love Jesus. The thought that I might be healed is a wonderful hope, but there are greater things that will be accomplished when we are obedient to the call to be *grounded and rooted in love.* And they will be accomplished when our faith is founded on a solid rock.

When "the vicissitudes of life" happen, we are able to overcome because of love.

Getting to the Wedding on Time

Living with ALS turns time into patterns of hope and despair. Announcements are received; dates are set; plans are made, while your expectation of reaching them is shrouded in the uncertainties of physical degeneration. Your hope of getting there is woven with despair that you won't. Each event is a milestone. They are lined up on the road ahead but don't try to see more than one at a time.

Two markers landed in my roadway in the first half of the year 2000. The first was set when our daughter, Karen, phoned from Sooke Harbor House in Victoria to tell us that she had just accepted a proposal of marriage from R.J. Shortly after, they set August 19 as their wedding date. While the creeping effects of muscle degeneration are even and consistent one never knows when the loss of strength will mean a buckling of the legs, the last switch of a toe or finger, or more dramatically still, the last suck of breath by the voluntary contraction of the diaphragm muscles. We measure our anticipations by days and weeks; months are gifts and half years and full years difficult to anticipate fully. So how did I anticipate that day when I might walk my daughter down the aisle? Would I be breathing without assistance? Would my petulant body spoil the road show by blowing all four tires three days before the party? Was I being perverse, negative, or morose? All of these could possibly happen but I was still full of hope that yet another milestone will be reached.

Logistical Difficulties

During the engagement period, my lung capacity dropped measurably but not dramatically. As a result I began to consistently take afternoon naps with my breathing assist machinery (called a BiPap) but was still able to breathe on my own for the balance of the day. The nuptials were to take place on the grounds of a bed and breakfast home owned by R.J.'s sister, Kathi, and her husband, Don. The five acre grounds and large colonial style house are located in the small rural community of Saltair on Vancouver Island, a one-and-a-half hour ferry ride and a one-hour drive from our home. This created logistical issues for us as we considered our accumulation of medical assist devices and special needs. But quickly the months moved by and it became clear that I would, indeed, ride my power chair down the aisle to tender my daughter's hand in marriage.

Early in the planning process, Lynne and I offered to perform the marriage ceremony and this suggestion was received with enthusiasm by both Karen and R.J. They had no church affiliation to draw from and warmed to the idea of not having to invite another body to the party that would involve both travel costs and honorarium, not to mention the possible two additional table settings. I asked one of our pastors, Paddy Ducklow, for copies of wedding vows and related material and some direction on how we would coordinate the legal elements of the marriage with the public service. He immediately emailed me a mass of data from which I was able to extract the basic wording of the "I do's" and wedding vows. I began to work on a short homily based on Psalm 19, a passage that was impressing itself upon me at the time, and which I thought I could twist into service.

On the issue of satisfying legal requirements Paddy casually suggested that we could sign documents before and after the wedding. We spent no time interpreting this suggested scenario until a week before the wedding when we went to Paddy for clarification and found that he would be on holidays. Paddy referred us to Rob DesCotes, one of the other pastors in the church, who was more than willing to take the matter on but was much less casual about the process. We had, by this time, arranged to have the entire bridal party meet at our home on the Wednesday before the wedding to sign documents, naively assuming that we could carry them to the event like draft documents, apply some finishing touches like the date, and mail of them in the next day. Not so fast, preacher boy. The authorized government agent must not only witness the marriage vows but also date them at the time. Sounds like a complete wedding.

So it was that on Wednesday, August 16, Karen and R.J. were wed legally by Rob before four legal witnesses and then on Saturday, August 19, were wed again, this time emotionally by Brian and Lynne Smith before 135 well-dressed witnesses. The bride arrived with her attendants at the second ceremony on a horse drawn buggy to the cheers of the assembled guests and was led down the aisle, formed by two rows of Gerbera daisies, by her father in his electrically powered chair.

The Faltering Proud Father of the Bride

Once settled in my place facing the guests with the descending grassy grounds and Gulf of Georgia as our backdrop, I asked them "Who gives this woman to be married to this man?" Then I quickly added my own startled response, "I do!" We had decided to start the ceremony with individual introductions of the bride and groom feeling that there were many in attendance who knew only one of them. R.J.'s brother-in-law, Lorne, gave a brief bio of him and I followed, introducing Karen, as follows:

I sit before you as a very proud father of this bride. Out of four children we only got one that could have become one and she has succeeded magnificently. My mind is filled with a blur of memories sandwiched between two white gowns. From a tiny flannel night dress to a wedding gown in 26 years and she did it hardly breaking a sweat. At least that's the impression she has left me with. She is no doubt thinking right now, "Sure, Dad, you were just not paying attention." And there would be some truth to that.

But I did pay enough attention to recognize some important things about her. She has an indomitable spirit that embraces everyone around her. She cares for the underdog, congratulates the winners, consoles the losers and can hang out joyously with any of them.

She has the ability to recognize and laugh uproariously at human oddity. But it is a laugh of identity not of ridicule.

She can sing a song on demand, compose a clever poem at the drop of a hat, describe her next two career goals during dessert, and be late for two events at the same time.

She can knock the cover off a softball, throw one like a

boy and be the sweetest, most gorgeous daughter anyone ever had. And she is mine.

But the time has come when I must give this complex package of feminine appeal away to another man. R.J., I proudly give Karen Marjorie Baker Smith to you to be your wife.

Then I slid into the actual ceremony with the following remarks:

Well, we have accomplished the remarkable feat of gathering this group of family and friends together on this site and have the two lovers standing before us. What's left to do but marry them? R.J. and Karen, you have invited us here to witness the transfiguration of your lives from man and woman into husband and wife. You have graciously asked me, your father and soon to be father-in-law, to help you accomplish that goal.

Never having carried out this function before I consulted with one of the pastors of our church. He emailed me four files filled with ceremonial invocations and masses of scripture readings related to marriage and love. I concluded that most of you have probably already attended several weddings in the past year and that therefore you have heard most of that already. I am neither pastor nor priest, only a faltering father with a desire to pass on some spiritual wisdom. So I have decided to simply offer some directives towards the source of wisdom rather than actually pass it on. To do that I turn to a Psalm written by King David over 2500 years ago. Its wisdom still stands.

"The heavens declare the glory of God; the skies proclaim the work of his hands.
Day after day they pour forth speech; night after night they display knowledge.
There is no speech or language where their voice is not heard.
Their voice goes out into all the earth, their words to the ends of the world. In the heavens he has pitched a tent for the sun, which is like a bridegroom coming forth from his pavilion, like a champion rejoicing to run his course.
It rises at one end of the heavens and makes its circuit to the other; nothing is hidden from its heat.
The law of the Lord is perfect, reviving the soul. The statutes of the Lord are trustworthy, making wise the simple.
The precepts of the Lord are right, giving joy to the heart. The commands of the Lord are radiant, giving light to the eyes.
The fear of the Lord is pure, enduring forever. The ordinances of the Lord are sure and altogether righteous.
They are more precious than gold, than much pure gold; they are sweeter than honey, than honey from the comb.
By them is your servant warned; in keeping them there is great reward.
Who can discern his errors? Forgive my hidden faults.
Keep your servant also from willful sins; may they not rule over me. Then will I be blameless, innocent of great transgression.
May the words of my mouth and the meditation of my heart be pleasing in your sight, O Lord, my Rock and my Redeemer" (Psalm 19:1–14).

Closing Comments

I have chosen this Psalm for our meditation because it directs us to the source of all wisdom, God. The first six verses tell us that the beauty, complexity and order of the universe are sufficient evidence for us to accept God's hand as the centre of our known world. No speech is required. The rising and setting sun, the feel of its heat, the sound of the wind and the brilliance of these daisies all tell us, without words, that God is there and he loves us. But all of this would be a waste if he had not placed us in the middle of this created world. And right now you, Karen and R.J., are in the middle of ours. He created us to be here and to praise him for what he has done.

Verses seven to eleven describe the second way in which we can know God and that is through his Word. The Scriptures are full of the rules for living and this Psalm describes eloquently the consequences and rewards of knowing them and following them. What I point you towards here is not familiar to this generation. One of the most enduring memories of my childhood was my grandmother, Karen's great-grandmother, using Scriptures to challenge my conduct. Twenty-five years later, when she was near the end of her life and we visited her with our young children she still had her Bible open on her bureau waiting for the opportune time to teach us her latest lesson. Now, three generations later, I am here to testify that she knew the source of wisdom. As I deal daily with the reality of the shortness of life I am drawn closer and closer to the Scriptures for comfort, peace and hope.

But please hear me; this is not just a book for weddings and funerals, for old women and dying men. This is the book for living life every day. This is your book for life because it leads us to Jesus.

This Psalm, as I have said, speaks first of creation and creation leads us to Jesus. The Scriptures themselves say that all things were created in him and for him. He is the Alpha and Omega, the beginning and the end.

Secondly, the Psalm speaks of statutes and words. Notice that this Psalm does not say; "Here are the rules, do them or else." Each line provides a comforting promise that results from understanding and doing. The truths and rules embodied in Scripture are freeing not condemning. Once again these truths are embodied in the person of Jesus himself. Scriptures say that the Word became flesh and dwelt among us. It is through his words that we learn to pray. His words in the gospels challenge us, comfort us, encourage us, free us and by his resurrection we are given new and eternal life. And we invite him here to be part of our wedding celebration as he was at the wedding in Cana of Galilee.

The Cost of Getting Married

In my review of the legal implications of marriage I concluded that there are three parts to the marriage mechanism. I list them in ascending order of cost. Firstly there is the sexual union. Done in the proper context this has no monetary cost.

Secondly, there is the legal marriage document. This costs $107.

Finally, and most importantly, is the public ceremony where the bride and groom make their vows in public. This generally costs between $15,000 and $30,000.

What is my point in listing these three elements in this way? Partly it's because I think in this quirky way. But more importantly I want to make a point about each.

First, there is the sexual union. In spite of the fact that our society it is attempting to turn sexuality into a recreational sport, God's intention is that it is the ultimate in our physical, emotional, and spiritual commitment to one another. The Bible says that the two become one flesh. Karen said to us the other day, "I'm so excited, I have a partner. He will always be there." And this vital part of marriage brings us back to the creation that we have talked about in Psalm 19. God has given us this gift of being able to access his creative power in the forming of new life. It is an awesome and mystical responsibility.

The second element is the legal contract. Even our society recognizes the sanctity of this institution. Karen and R.J. chose to sign that contract with Carla and Owen as witnesses prior to this ceremony so that their public vows would be the final element sealing their marriage covenant. But the legal contract is an indication that society affirms the sanctity of it.

Finally, we sanctify marriage by making public vows in the presence of God. In doing so we add the most important element—that of the covenant that Karen and R.J. make between themselves and God in the presence of those who will support them and care for them in the passage of life. One of my favourite books in the Bible is Ecclesiastes. One of its wise statements is, "Though one may be overpowered, two can defend themselves. A cord of three strands is not quickly broken" (4:12). I like to think of this passage in relation to the marriage covenant. Karen's comment about partnership speaks to the issue of the second part where two people stand up for each other. The third strand is their invitation to God to join with them in this covenant which is formed by the vows they are about to make.

I want to take us back to the last verse of this Psalm which is a prayer that if followed will safeguard this marriage covenant. It goes like this. "May the words of my mouth and the meditation of my heart be pleasing in your sight, O LORD, my Rock and my Redeemer." R.J. and Karen, if your hearts and minds are set on pleasing God you will always please each other. And God's way is easily found—found in the speechless grandeur of our universe, in the written word of Scripture and in your hearts and minds planted by his Spirit.

Lynne followed my talk with a brief explanation of each of the vows the couple were about to invoke. Then I read the marital pledge to each of them, to which they enthusiastically replied, "I do." The vows and the exchanging of rings rounded out the formalities and we announced them as husband and the wife, Mr. and Mrs. R.J. Parry. Then the celebration began.

The bride and groom were swept away in the horse drawn carriage for a ceremonial excursion from the wedding to the reception. Since both were being held at the same location it involved a ride out the driveway, through a neighbour's property, and back. In that time the chairs were moved to the marquee where the tables were being set for dinner.

Toasts and talks took place, effectively organized by the M.C.s, Kyle and Craig Smith, the bride's two oldest brothers. The trigger for prompting a bridal kiss was the performance of a "stupid human trick." Several were performed including the bride's aunt touching her tongue to the nose.

But the touching highlights included a sensitive but amusing toast to the bride by her brother, Fraser. Then parts of a letter written by Karen's mother prior to her death in

1994 were read by Karen's friend, Iris. Finally there was a moving tribute to my loving bride, Lynne, by the bride of the hour who expressed, on behalf of all her siblings, the great gratitude they feel for such a loving person to have entered the lives of both their father and themselves.

Getting to Another Wedding on Time

As I mentioned earlier there were two milestone events lined up on the road. The first was the wedding of my daughter. Then in May our son Kyle and his wife Leslie advised us that the expected date of the birth of our first grandchild is to be December 4. As I was heading to another wedding celebration—the marriage supper of the Lamb in the new heaven and new earth (Revelation 19)—I was not sure I would be present to see my first grandchild.

June 24, 2000

To my first grandchild,

It is several weeks now since your mom and dad told us that our first potential grandchild was forming in your mother's womb. We are all cautious about getting too excited because the first time that a tiny life began to form there it died before it was very big. You are almost four months in growing and we all hope we will see you as a living, breathing, healthy baby in early December.

The reason I am writing this message to you is that I may not be here when you come. By the time you read this you will already have heard about me and seen pictures so I don't need to explain why this may be the case. Even if I do see you and have the opportunity of holding you in my arms it is unlikely that you will know me other than from what you are told or from what I have written. If I am able to see you and hold you it will be a great blessing to me but not to see you grow through your childhood will be an immeasurable sorrow.

One milestone passed; another almost certain to be missed.

Closing Comments

I cannot speak genuinely or deeply of resurrection
except I speak the same of death
and the sin that engendered death. That I can
speak accurately of death without
despairing is hardly melancholic. It is liberty—
and victory ("O Death, where is thy sting?").

Walter Wangerin, Jr.

I think a really big issue for some people is the psychological one of letting go of the idea that we can still do it. When you finally give in and say, "I can't walk," getting into a chair makes life much more liveable. My breathing is so low that it exhausts me just to stand in front of my chair and take a pee but I can still go for long walks with my wife and move around my apartment freely.

Wally Eggert sent me an email. I delayed answering and then wrote:

Sorry to take so long in reply. I have actually composed a number of messages to you from my chair, thoughts which have elicited mysterious tears of nostalgia and regret. Why is it that the simple kind words of a friend can turn my insides to mush? Sometimes there is just too much history to bear—especially when separation and radical change breaks the string. I really do miss contact with you.

Of course, your comments about kids tweaks both of the emotional keys mentioned above but not often enough do my anxieties move my spirit to prayer.

You would think that as my physical activities become restricted the time left for reflection would naturally lead to such activity. But I find it no easier. In the face of the internal struggles I fear becoming preoccupied with myself. And what an awful conclusion that would be.

And later I wrote to Dana Armerding, Jenny's son, who also uses a power chair.

Hi Dana,

Thank you for the picture but you should stop snapping your fingers. Scientific research has determined that there is a direct relationship between finger snapping and teeth falling out. Apparently when you snap your fingers the vibration goes all the way up your arm, through your shoulder, into your neck, then into your jawbone and right into the roots of your teeth. Then they just fall out. The only way to keep your teeth from falling out when you snap your fingers is to always hold your left big toe with your other hand while you are snapping your fingers. This stops the vibration. You look kind of funny doing it but at least you keep your teeth. It's an awful nuisance waiting for new teeth to grow back in.

When we have stopped being so busy we may well come down to visit you. Some time ago we took my chair on an airplane when we went to Toronto. They bent my head-rest but we got it fixed. I like going to the park with you and I wish we could do it more often. I have never gone riding in the park with someone with a missing tooth but I guess it could be done.

Please say happy birthday to Malcolm for me. I love you, too. Also your mom and Malcolm, but maybe you a bit more.... But don't tell them that.

Love,
Brian.

I am still determined to be content.

During this last year I have progressed from scooter to power chair. My ability to walk has been reduced to a dozen steps, partly due to the problem of balance, but more from lack of energy. Muscles continue to atrophy and my respiration level is below 30 percent. But somehow we feel fortunate when we are aware of other ungrateful recipients of this malady where the disease progresses at a faster rate. One thing we have learned as we cope with this disease is that everyone's experience is different.

In our case we are thankful that our needs to date have been manageable without an audible scream for help. Our principal needs have been in the area of handyman help and our current list of acknowledgements includes: Mike Nichols and Jake Penner (bookcase construction), Gord Taylor (anything and whenever needed) and Ralph Bagshaw (finding an adjustable bed). Being dependent can be very humbling but most of all I feel enveloped in the love of other people. I used to look at things I had made with great personal pride. Now I look at something that is made *for* me and am reminded of God's love for me through other people. So maybe in the end this is much better.

I was speaking of "our" needs. But we are really talking about my needs and they are met by one person. She faces them virtually 24 hours a day. She is my feet, my hands, my encourager, my personal live-in saint. She is my wife.

Probably I am too wrapped up in the damned inconvenience of this thing to think much about the death part. When I do think of it I counter it with the blessings of the life I have lived. Somehow I relate the logic of it to a length of life. So when I watch Morrie die (in the film "Tuesdays with Morrie," about the sociology professor who died of the same disease), I think, "Well, you're 78; that's a pretty long life and you have to die of something." On the other hand I look at a couple of guys in our support group who are twenty years younger than I am and think, "That's a major bummer compared with me; I had a pretty good run of it."

Of course, I didn't want Morrie to die either and I shed tears at several points in the film—mainly when I could identify with his feelings. His comment about self-pity is right on. You wake up to it every day and you have to shuck it off, tell yourself it's the way it is and get on with it. Sometimes though, when I am alone, I just break down and cry about it. It always seems like self-pity but maybe it is more like anguish. Suddenly I just dry up and generally it feels good. But we can always console ourselves by the fact that Jesus did it all, including the cries of anguish.

Lately, I have had a few fits of minor depression when I face the limits of my life. This disease isolates one from so much. I would like to think that I still have some usefulness. But I must find ways of being useful outside of areas that I normally was productive in.

Sometimes I feel sorry for myself. But it doesn't do much good. I think most of the time I accept the gift of tranquility as an adequate offset to all the activity and running around that I am missing. The shortness of life is something we all should face every day and do the most with what we have today. Because of my condition I spend time wondering what the transition will be between this life and the next. It is a wonderful mystery, and one which at times I even doubt. But in the end I rely on the scriptural promises and my limited understanding of the new creation which only a loving God could have imagined. What do we have without Jesus, "the radiance of God's glory and the exact representation of his being"?

After we visited the respirologist today we visited an ALS friend at Vancouver General Hospital who went on a respirator just before Christmas and still is not out of the hospital from various complications. If I continue to do well with my speaking ability and have some arm and leg mobility I think I will continue as I am. But if I were to find myself in the condition that he appears to be in I think I would rally my troops around and say my farewells. There are too many scriptural images of life with the everlasting Father and Son for me to want to endure the effort that we would all need to exert for me to cling to the bottom (or is it the top?) rung of this earthly ladder.

But how do I really know what I would do? What is it that makes us want to hang on so hard?

Well, I know some reasons... one just came and kissed me.

Closing Comments

The first time I laid eyes on Brian was in late September, five years ago. I was drawn to him from that moment, and more amazingly, he to me. Our spirits danced with delight at all the possibilities that lay before us. But even then, although we did not know it, he was sick. Soon the dancing would turn for a brief moment to mourning. Brief, because Brian allowed us to keep dancing. He wanted his living while dying to enrich the lives of all he knew and who came to know him. He wanted people to see Jesus in him. He did this. He understood that dancing and mourning are the stuff of life, of life that is full and rich.

Early in the morning of October 4, 2000, I reached over to touch him as I had done what seems like hundreds of times that night. He was peaceful. It took me a few minutes to realize that his earthly journey was over and that he was now dancing in the presence of the Lord. He had reached the destination he so longed for. The years have been few but the dancing far overshadowed the mourning. We lived and now even more poignantly, dwell, in the shelter of the Most High. We rest in the shadow of the Almighty.

My pilgrimage continues. But thanks to Brian I have a few more tools for the journey. Love, faithfulness, children and grandchildren, possibility.

Thank you my love,
Lynne

Eulogy for Brian Smith
April 28, 1940–October 4, 2000

By Wally Eggert
October 10, 2000
West Vancouver Baptist Church

I can't help being struck by the irony and ambivalence of the moment. We have feelings of sadness and loss, feelings of grief and heaviness. Yet, I think Brian, while accepting our tears and anguish, would want us to change our focus—from tears of sadness to tears of laughter, from anguish and grief to inner peace and joy. He would want us to dwell, not on our loss, but on *who* and *what* we still have. He would want us to *use this time* to not only focus on him, but to look within and gain a new appreciation of the people in our lives.

The irony and ambivalence extends to a struggle with what to say of him. We would come into his presence expecting to laugh, expecting to be entertained with a joke, a skit, or a surprise visit from one of his many characters, because, Brian was, to quote Lynne, "a very funny guy; and such a handsome one at that."

Brian Loved Life

But, that's not all that Brian was. He was a complex person.

He was an analyst, a critic, and of late a serious and reflective writer. He was an intellectual and a philosopher of sorts, an athlete, a carpenter, a businessman, entrepreneur and an accountant. He would much rather have been in a shop, on a job site or on the beach interacting with people, than in the office, behind a desk, crunching numbers.

Think of it—an intelligent, risk-taking, artistic, accountant, who loved to use a chain saw and pound nails. Now that could be dangerous—and it was.

We know so much of Brian the comedian. However, I am reminded of Brian the man of faith and hope, who sought and found a reason for the hope that was within him. He became more heavenly minded but he *so* loved to live life in the here and now. Life was too short for Brian.

I first met Brian about 40 years ago playing touch football. He loved sports—golf, fishing, water-skiing, tennis, and hockey at 2:00 a.m. with a bunch of guys who couldn't skate or afford ice at a reasonable time of the day. We use to say while driving to the rink, what are we doing this for? We simply loved it.

Brian loved to live his life in community. He was not afraid to get close to people, to get involved with us; to offer an empathic ear; to self-disclose his own imperfections and difficulties (and he endured more than his share). He met so many of us where we are most vulnerable. His clients, his sister Andrea tells me, talk, *not so much* about the great accountant he was, but what a great man he was. He didn't see them as business associates; he got involved personally because he cared for people. He had compassion for family, friends, neighbors, campers, and clients alike. He drew people to himself, embracing and accepting without judgement.

So when I think of this wonderfully complex, yet

uncomplicated friend, who loved us, who loved life and now is taken from us, I want to brood, not laugh. The temptation for this self-indulgence is there. Brian experienced it too.

He wrote:

> *In spite of great intentions to keep on the right track we often get derailed and the sense of loss that I have felt as my physical state deteriorates and I watch people doing all the physical activities I have enjoyed, sends me into my lowest spots.*

But let's not go there yet.

Brian the Comedian

We could always count on Brian to come up with something to make us laugh, at camp, or at a wedding, at an anniversary, birthday, or block party. We expected him to perform. When arriving at one of these events, I wanted to sit at his table so as not to miss a single joke.

If he wasn't telling a joke, he wanted to hear one. Two weeks ago, when visiting with him and others, he said, "Wally, tell the one about the frog that you emailed the other day." I began, and of course left out a point critical to the delivery of the punch line. Brian graciously filled in the gap and then laughed as if it was the first time he had heard it.

Brian studied stand-up comedians, their material and routines, adapting and creating his own unique style and characters. He blended his ability to ad lib with the discipline of planning and preparation.

We will never forget Brian's characters and their routines—the surprise entries and heroic deeds as Superman. Then there were his extraordinary academic lectures on almost any topic as Dr. Broomfarkel. And the man of amazing feats and few words, Dr. Noid. Noid provided his audiences with bizarre demonstrations of his research findings.

Once at a Pioneer Family Camp, Dr Noid, after extensive study of the growth of hair on babies, claimed he could make hair appear on the head of a bald camper.

His skeptical interviewer asked Dr. Noid, "You do that?"

"YEEESSHH," said Noid.

"Can you show us"? asked the interviewer.

"YEEESSHH," replied Noid.

"Well show us then," urged the impatient interviewer.

"YEEESSHH," replied Noid .

Dr. Noid, without a word, whipped out a pair of scissors, cut a lock of hair from the head of a young camper and pasted it on the bald camper's head and proudly said,

"SEEEEE—HAAAIRRRR."

Incensed, the camp manager rushed to the aid of the young de-locked camper, grabbed Dr. Noid, and just as he was about to whack him, Dr Noid was heard to say,

"YOU DON'T KNOW WHO YOU ARE DEALING WITH."

Shedding his outer garments, Noid transformed to Superman, and with a *Biff!* a *Bam!* and a *Pow!* disposed of the camp manager, to the delight and glee of children and adults alike.

The anticipation of seeing one of Brian's characters created an image that made us laugh. Brian would simply appear in character, stretching his 6'4" frame to at least 6'8", stand stoically and wait for the gales of laughter to subside. These characters grew on us, like we knew them as real people.

Petra (my daughter) recalls, "When I was a little girl and first saw Superman at Pioneer Pacific, I knew it was Brian. Superman engaged in a tug-of-war (it was Superman against all the men and boys in camp), the rope extending across the pool, and Superman pulled all of the opposition into the water. She said, "I knew it was fake, but I believed that he was Superman and that he really did that," as did so many other little campers.

Brian was in Victoria and came to Lambrick Park Church with us. A little boy, who had been to family camp that very summer, saw Brian from some distance. With eyes as wide as saucers, the boy, was heard to say, "*Look Mommy, there is Superman!*" People turned to see who he was looking at. They could not see what the little boy saw.

Brian knew how to play *let's pretend* until we thought it was real.

I'm looking forward to some of the Brian "classics," such as The Made by Pioneer Video Productions—*Superman—Super-Pee* (or was it called Forest Dump?). I want to hear the story of Brian upstaging the Crash Test Dummies performance at the Commodore as they were singing their hit—*Superman's Song*—and Brian jumping on the stage and, sporting his Superman costume, leaping into the crowd, his cape trailing behind as the people passed him along overhead. I want to hear it again, Kyle. You were there. I want to hear it at least once a year for the rest of my life.

But Brian wasn't pretending when he fell in love with Lynne. It was for real and our little children—who loved to believe in Superman, now young adults—saw him fall in love with Lynne. It happened right in front of us and it was great. It is indeed a real love story, beautiful, with drama, romance, and the miraculous (absolutely no comparison to the heroic feats of Superman).

Brian was so transparent to our children and they loved him. Two of our sons, David and John, lived with Brian and

Barb for a time. This upright man has influenced them, along with Petra and Joe, *and many of your kids*, for so much that was good and true.

He sent an email to Corinne, David's wife, the other day:

> *Congratulations on the use of your body for the procreation of the human race.*

Brian the Spiritual Leader

In the early '70s, several families, including Brian and Barb and their kids, all of us living in North Van, started a home church. This is when I saw Brian's hunger for a deeper understanding of the Scriptures. He asked penetrating questions, encouraging critical thought and serious study. He wanted the Scriptures to be a guide for our real life problems and issues. While he honored his Christian family heritage he worked at making his faith *personal and acquired,* as opposed to simply *induced.*

Brian was working out his own salvation while accepting the fact that *God was at work in him.* He knew he was a sinner saved by grace. He also recognized his role in the process and he gave himself to it.

Brian became *a spiritual leader and mentor*, although he would never say that. He began to teach and lead Bible Studies sharing not so much the answers but the better questions. He became an elder in his church. Brian continued to grow spiritually until the end. His learning curve took another steep incline in these last four years with Lynne.

Brian had every reason to become cynical, bitter and pessimistic. But it was his hope that was infectious. It was grounded in his conviction that the Jesus of the New Testament was real. It *"was grounded in the historic Christ-event"* (Henri Nouwen). He believed that Jesus was a real human being, who lived and died here on earth for our redemption. It was clear to Brian that the Jesus who loved us and humbled himself even unto death was worthy of his love. Brian loved God. And by following Christ, Brian knew he would have new life.

In a recent email, he wrote:

> *I have been reading in first John Chapter 5, where, we see that even our ability to* ***overcome*** *is wrapped up in love.*
>
> *"Verse 3, Loving God means doing what He tells us to do, and really, that isn't hard at all; v. 4, for every child of God can obey him defeating sin and evil pleasure by trusting Christ to help.... v. 5, But who could possibly fight and win this battle except by believing that Jesus is truly the Son of God?"*
>
> *It really is quite simple, isn't it Wally?*

Brian was certain that he was surrounded by God's love. He wrote:

> *Another comfort for me, both in endurance and in anticipating what is to come, is a daily reading in the Psalms. Today I read the following. The images are full of security:*
>
> *"Those who trust in the Lord are steady like Mount Zion, unmoved by any circumstance, enduring forever. Just as the mountains surround and protect Jerusalem, so the LORD surrounds his people. He always has and always will" (Psalm 125).*

So Brian wanted us to take comfort in the fact that he knew and trusted in God. He wrote:

> *I was to discover that my children would lose both their parents prematurely... when this happens prematurely I need to reassure others, particularly my children, that I am content, that my destination is set, and that my work is done.*

One of the last things Brian said to me was this:

> *I live with the tension between here and there and sometimes I'd rather be there.*

You *know* that he was thinking of heaven and the hereafter. He even asked many of you what you thought heaven would be like. I think he made light of your views of heaven at his sixtieth birthday party to ease the tension. He wanted to live. He loved being with us. We will remember him most for his love. You could see it in his eyes. So, he wanted this cup to pass. He sought understanding by looking to Jesus.

He wrote:

> *I know that Jesus was tempted in all ways that I am and I know that he too sought relief by calling out to have "this cup" taken from him.*

Brian, Part of the Eternal Solution

Even when he was in serious trouble, near to the end, Brian was concerned not so much for himself as he was for others. He visited children confined to wheelchairs. He took them for "walks, so to speak," and without patronizing, showed his compassion and humor. He could wiggle his ears to the end. They loved him.

And Lynne. Lynne will miss her big handsome Brian whom she loved so dearly. When I asked him, how should we pray, he wrote:

> *And pray for Lynne. She is the one to needs the stamina for two. She fulfills all of the practical requirements of this thing at this time, but the time will come when help will be needed. Today I wrote in my journal "Fraser leaves Saturday and plans to be up there for six months. So great for him but not something I like thinking about. I feel the compression of time and sometimes it fills me with a sweet sort of sorrow." The time I spend with any of them (Kyle and Leslie, Craig and Julia, Karen and R.J.) now seems so valuable and this is a subtracted chunk against the youngest of the brood (Fraser). Sorry, I think I pick on you to dump this stuff....*

What a privilege to be dumped on by Brian. He was always so willing to hear me dump on him. I'm going to miss him.

Finally, Brian wrote:

> *Enough for now. Thank you for the memories, both those we currently enjoy and the ones we are about to create. Thank you for being part of the eternal solution.*

There is pain and sorrow to bear, but, in time, the warmth of our memories will comfort us. Brian enriched our lives immeasurably.

He gave us a profound wit from which much laughter came.

He gave us a good heart from which compassion and love came.

He gave us his friendship, which gave us a new appreciation for each other.

He gave us deep spiritual leadership which strengthened our hope and faith.

He demonstrated *a part of the eternal solution,* which gives us peace and joy.

Brian wrote:

> *Only one man knew the source and reason for his suffering. "Surely he took up our infirmities and carried our sorrows, yet we thought he was punished by God, smitten by him, and afflicted, But He was pierced for our transgressions, He was crushed for our iniquities" (Isaiah 53: 4–5). So instead of finding reason, we find redemption. And to find comfort I look to his affliction.*

We thank God that Brian has been redeemed—into the arms of Jesus.

Nice going, Brian. We love you and miss you.

At the Graveside

By Graeme Smith

Some years ago at one of several funerals I attended over a relatively short period of time, it occurred to me during the eulogy that there was something inherently false about celebrating a loved one's entrance into eternity solely in terms of praise and commendation and ignoring the half of the whole person that we knew, whose less than admirable characteristics we endured, reproached or suffered; the half of the person for which presumably eternity really meant a sunrise—promised healing and release. I remember sharing this with Brian and he, as usual, instantly understood what I was struggling to give words to, and we talked about it at some length. We ultimately concluded that whatever merits my insight had it would take a very deft touch indeed to pull it off in a funeral without coming off as mean and ill-spirited. I certainly lack that touch but I do want to attempt to share with you something of my perception of who Brian was, as a whole person, and at the same time, share with you what I feel I can say, with some confidence, two brothers think awaits us at the crossroad of life and death and time and eternity.

Over the past few weeks I have thought a lot about the nature of my relationship with my brother. "Close" was the first word that came to mind. But my ready answer prompted me to ask myself how I would define "close." Over the past 40-plus years of our adult life I could count on one hand the number of times he and I had done anything together as brothers. We did have an unusually common mind on almost anything we ever talked about when we did get together, but what I think more than anything defined our closeness was our shared conviction that we were failures.

Now, nobody who knew Brian would call him a failure. When five or six hundred people show up at your funeral you must have been remarkably successful at something! But how others view us and how we view ourselves are two quite separate things. What we imagine others think of us and what they actually do think of us are equally sure to be quite different. And these differences are almost certain to break along all kinds of complex and even contradictory lines. At the root of this phenomenon is what Christian theology defines as original sin, but since that is a concept that is commonly misunderstood (and we have no time here to try to clarify it) I will attempt to describe this root problem in terms of the "broken self."

From the very beginning, our emerging self-consciousness is characterized by brokenness. The conflict between what we want and what our parents want for us begins in infancy—and that battle waged on the emotional field of desire for parental approval produces the broken self. As we grow older this self-image becomes increasingly complex. Awareness of physical shortcomings, emotional inadequacies, intellectual deficiencies, and habits and character flaws that seem to have genetic inevitability and permanence all contribute to the makeup of our broken selves. Perhaps equally important the inadequacies and failures of parents, siblings, and others who made up our childhood environment have their own inevitable destructive impact on us. And we live out our lives making strenuous, but largely ineffectual, efforts to compensate for or to conceal this flawed self-image either from ourselves or others. We all struggle with this to varying degrees of success. The few who appear to be unencumbered with such feelings of inadequacy more or less comprise those who "make history" in small ways and large. At the other end are those who are paralyzed by their brokenness and spend their days dumpster-diving and pushing shopping carts full of our refuse. The vast majority of us, however, muddle along as best we can, accompanied by our light and dark angels of hope and despair. Brian was one of us.

My brother as you all know was a very funny guy, but you might not have been aware that his wry, ironic, sometimes even sardonic sense of humour had its roots in his own experiences of frustration and failure. I think at heart he was a clown in the tradition of the legendary Emmett Kelly, the circus clown with the sad face making children laugh. There was often something in Brian's comic performances which transcended the laughter and touched something sadder and much deeper in our experiences together as human beings, that exposed the struggle of our broken selves. His Crash Test Dummies concert stage crashing performance took place during the final tortuous weeks of Barbara Jean's life when he confessed to me that his sense of inadequacy, confusion and fear threatened to overwhelm him and he felt he had to do something to break the spell of despair, and what better way to do that than to don the Superman persona.

Somehow the staged irony of the Superman cape and his own sense of helplessness in the face of his impending loss was a form of therapy for his soul that must have put a smile on the face of God himself, who I am sure understood it better than Brian did.

I was not present for that appearance of Superman, but I was present for another appearance that will remain indelibly imprinted on my memory more for what it represented than for the comic moment itself. When Brian appeared at his sixtieth birthday party in his superman costume and his electric wheel chair, it struck me that there could have been no better metaphor than that for his whole life. The lifelong handicap of his inborn pessimism and sense of failure never thwarted his attempts "to leap tall buildings in a single bound." His spirit always longed to be "up, up, and away!" and I think in his illness the more his body mocked him the more his spirit soared. Now of course his Master has taken him "up, up, and away" to a whole other realm!

Had Brian only his humour to aid him in his struggle with the broken self he would never have become the man we have honoured these past two days. As a follower of Jesus he had within reach and touch the ultimate antidote for the broken self—the unconditional love of Jesus.

I don't know about each of you who follows Jesus, but I have found, and I know this was true for Brian, that the efficacy of that divine love is fleeting. We only grasp enough of it to sustain the conviction that it is real and reinforce the hope that one day we will experience its full resurrection power. There are many who make bold statements about how we can realize it in the here and now, but ironically these promises are usually accompanied by "conditions." I think in the end, it is Jesus who reaches out and grants us those moments of release and freedom; but the reasons and timing are known only to him.

On the morning of Brian's death, shortly after the undertakers had taken his body away, I sat between Lynn and Craig, and Craig mused about what his father was doing at that moment. Lynn quickly responded that he was breathing deeply and freely, inhaling and exhaling without encumbrance. In these reflective moments the dominant feeling I am experiencing is not grief but rather envy. Now finally my brother can breathe, without hindrance, the divine air of unconditional love. When the Lord of the Universe, face to face, cast those eyes of love on Brian, the spell of his broken self was broken forever and now he is soaring in ways we can't even dream of.